On Depression

On Depression

Drugs, Diagnosis,

and Despair

in the Modern World

NASSIR GHAEMI

The Johns Hopkins University Press
Baltimore

The Johns Hopkins University Press
2715 North Charles Street
Baltimore, Maryland 21218-4363
www.press.jhu.edu

Library of Congress Cataloging-in-Publication Data

Ghaemi, Nassir.
    On depression. drugs, diagnosis, and despair in the modern world / Nassir
Ghaemi.
        p. ; cm.
    Includes bibliographical references and index.
    ISBN 978-1-4214-0933-7 (hardcover. alk.paper) — ISBN 1-4214-0933-X
(hardcover. alk. paper) — ISBN 978-1-4214-0934-4 (electronic) — ISBN 1-4214-
0934-8 (electronic)
    I. Title.
    [DNLM.   1. Depression—psychology.   2. Antidepressive
Agents.   3. Depressive Disorder—diagnosis.   4. Depressive Disorder—drug
therapy.   5. Diagnostic Errors.   6. Existentialism. WM 171. 5]
    616. 85′27—dc23   2012036893

A catalog record for this book is available from the British Library.

*Special discounts are available for bulk purchases of this book. For more information,
please contact Special Sales at 410-516-6936 or specialsales@press.jhu.edu.*

To Dr. Frederick K. Goodwin
and to Dr. Athanasios Koukopoulos

What was man?
In what part of his conversing,
of his laughter and whistling,
in which of his chemical movements
lived the indestructible,
the enduring,
the living?

PABLO NERUDA

I intended to write a book about happiness, but as I got into the topic I realized that I couldn't do so unless I also wrote about despair, and even depression, which also entailed discussing mania. So this is a book about what it means to have depression or bipolar illness and what it means to experience despair or happiness. I critique some views that I think are mistaken in these debates, and I explore those thinkers, especially from the existential tradition in psychiatry and psychology, whose wisdom needs to be heard.

Nietzsche said he loves only that which is written in blood. This book is an attempt to discover the meanings of depression and mania, not in a merely abstract sense, but with the insights, hard won and written in blood, of those whom I see and try to treat daily and of those who have taught me, in person and in books.

I   Entrance

For years I was unhappy, consciously and deliberately . . . so that I isolated myself more and more, undertook less and less. . . . The misery and solitude and apathy and sneers were the elements of an index of superiority and guaranteed the feeling of arrogant "otherness.". . . It was not until that way of living, or rather negation of living, developed such terrifying physical symptoms that it could no longer be pursued that I became aware of anything morbid in myself. In short, if the heart had not put the fear of death into me I would be still boozing and sneering and lounging around and feeling that I was too good for anything else.

SAMUEL BECKETT

CHAPTER 1

Lives of Quiet Desperation

THE MOST SALIENT FEATURE of our world is that God is dead. Or at least he appears to be dead. Perhaps he is on life support. Or maybe he has become an embalmed version of what he once was, appearing lifelike, but really dead. Nietzsche, formally and most famously, pronounced God dead. But perhaps the truth is closer to what Emerson said, less famously, half a century earlier: we live *as if* God were dead.

To many, the world is a flat and soulless place. It is a land in which to despair, a land for the already dead, pretending to be alive. To say that God is dead is to say that the spiritual impulse that once drove mankind has petered out. God inspired not just his believers but Voltaire in his unbelief and Marx in his messianism. God is dead because hope has died, because the world has become meaningless, because the ideals of the Enlightenment perished in gas chambers.

In a word, we are living in a postmodern world where nothing is true and nothing is false; the rational response to such a world is despair. Most of us don't despair, though, because we think we don't know what it means to say that the world is postmodern and God is dead. In fact, we know it so well—that the world is postmodern and God is dead—that we aren't conscious of what we know.

SOME DIVIDE THE WESTERN mind arbitrarily into three epochs: the premodern, the modern, and the postmodern. The premodern age was when God was alive: the West believed in the Lord, either through the ascendancy of Christendom, or even before, through the deities of Roman, Greek, and other religions. The world had order and law and meaning, all divinely ordained, sent to humans through books of revelation and enacted through the divine right of kings. This was, intellectually, the Garden of Eden of mankind. The universe was, one might argue, a much kinder and gentler place, intellectually, in the medieval era than it later became.

The modern era began when Europeans, inspired by Islamic thinkers (themselves rediscoverers of Greece and Rome), began to doubt the laws of God and man. The established order was put to the test of Reason, and Reason was seen as superior to Revelation or power. First in Italy—later in France and England and eventually in Germany and America—the revolution of Reason swept the West. God was taken ill. He was not dead yet, but he had lost his personal power. He had become subservient to Reason, needed to start the world in motion at the beginning of time but no longer serving active purposes in the lives of men. The American Founding Fathers invoked his name but always within the confines of rational thought. God had become sicklied o'er with the pale cast of thought (as Shakespeare's Hamlet put it)—but he still breathed.

The new spirit of Reason, and the old spirit of Revelation, coexisted for a while, but then began to conflict more directly after Darwin seemed to disprove the word of God, and, by the end of the nineteenth century, it became clear that the West was entering a new era. God was losing the battle with Reason, and eventually, as Emerson and Nietzsche and a few others noticed, God lost.

He died.

We entered the postmodern era, which we might date as beginning in the year 1900, when Nietzsche himself died after years of chronic insanity and later dementia.

Nietzsche was both the prophet and the critic of this postmodern world. He saw the harm of the premodern mind; life was placid mentally, but it was torture physically. God's rule in the mind was benign, but in the real world, men killed and slaughtered and died needlessly in his name. In the modern era, the reverse had happened: physical existence had improved; lives were more often saved than lost as science progressed; but mentally, mankind suffered great torture. It no longer knew what to believe; it had not yet let go of God, but it could no longer accept his word as final either. Nietzsche approved of the new mental freedom, even if it produced pain; the anesthesia of intellectual submission to God was not worth it. Truth was to be preferred. Still, he also wondered whether something had been lost with the end of the physical conflicts and challenges of the past. When life became safe and predictable and secure, had humanity lost something essential to being human?

To explain this dilemma, Nietzsche set up the antimony of two kinds of persons: the Superman and the Last Man, which I'll explain next.

HERE IS OUR DILEMMA in the Western world today: We are a hopeless and cynical people, and we think we are beacons of happiness. We have given up on the noble and the ideal, but we think our absence of ideals is noble. We think we are great countries, exporting the best values all over the world, yet we have lost our own values; we don't measure up to the greatness of our own forefathers.

We are, in Nietzsche's phrasing, Last Men, who think they are Supermen.

Nietzsche writes his thoughts on this topic in the epic genre, putting his words in that of the hero of his story, the Persian prophet Zarathustra, who comes upon the people of his age and sees that they have declined. He looks about him and tries to show his decadent people that they have fallen away from what was best in them. He sees that they have reached the end of their cultural existence, that they are the last men of their history.

"Alas," Zarathustra says, "the time of the most despicable is coming, he that is no longer able to despise himself. Behold, I show you the *last man*" (italics in original).

The Last Man is a creature of the postmodern world; he has given up the comfort of faith, and he has taken the efforts of Reason to be illusion. He is left with nothing but the self-satisfied feeling that he knows better than the believers and the rationalists. What he knows, however, is only that there is nothing to know. The content of his being is only negation—the negation of others, the refusal to stand up for anything, the disbelief in all except his own right to disbelieve. This is the American teenager within each one of us: a pure relativism that knows little and thinks that there is little to know.

Yet, except for the teenager himself, we do not usually state the beliefs of the Last Man so bluntly. Indeed, as we grow up, we do not think we are Last Men. Rather, we think we have achieved something greater, something Nietzsche wanted to achieve, what he called Superman.

Here is Nietzsche's version of human history: Man was once Man, pure and simple, but Man evolved into Master and Slave, and from those two types, Man then degenerated into the Last Man; and now his only way out is to become Superman.

Ubermensch is the German, which can also be translated "Overman." Superman connotes the comic hero, the movie screen hunk, flying across the big city, greater, much greater, than the average man. But perhaps even the comic myth contains within it the seed of Nietzsche's insight. For Superman is also Clark Kent; not only is he superhuman, he is human. Or perhaps he shows that the two can be the same: that what is human can be superhuman.

The word Overman gives the connotation that Nietzsche might have been seeking: to overcome man as he has become, to become more than the Last Man, to put all of them behind—the Last Man, the Master, the Slave. Man is not just one thing; there is no essence to him; so Man can change, and the Overman would be the next change, the next step beyond the Last Man, toward something better and greater than this most despicable version of humankind.

NIETZSCHE IS UNJUSTLY CARICATURED in the notion of a will to power. He is seen as simply exalting power over right, strength as the source of morality. This view collapses in the public mind with the atrocious use of Nietzschean terms by the German Nazi regime. Yet

Nietzsche's concept of power and morality was ambivalent; he characterized it as "the Roman Caesar with Christ's soul." Frequently I have laughed, Nietzsche makes Zarathustra say, at the weaklings who thought themselves good, because they had no power to be bad. They had no claws and forsook eating meat. Nietzsche wants us to be strong, and *then* to be good, not to pretend that our weakness represents goodness. The Last Man is weak and bad but pretends he is good; the Overman is to be strong and good and needs no pretension. Precisely because I deem you capable of all evil, Nietzsche says to those whom he wants to become Overmen, I demand the good from you.

This is rational. One cannot be held responsible for being a certain way, unless one is capable of being another way. In philosophical terms, agency precedes responsibility. Most of us know this when we think about evil: If we blame someone for a crime, it is because we think he could have avoided committing it. Indeed, if one is completely insane, and thus not able to act otherwise, we do not ascribe guilt. Nietzsche is arguing that the same logic holds for doing good: If we praise someone for goodness, it has to be because that person could have done something bad instead. This is why one has to be strong first, before one can be good; one has to be capable of evil in order to do good.

NIETZSCHE BECAME THE FAVORITE philosopher of a school of thought that has come to be called, generically, postmodernism. Its leading figures tend to be French (like Michel Foucault and Jacques Derrida), but there are also some Germans (Martin Heidegger and his followers).

Postmodernism isn't just a philosophy, though; it is a cultural movement, with impact in the arts, literature, social sciences—and even medicine and psychiatry, as we'll see.

A definition first:

Postmodernism is the notion that the "modernist" goal of discovering the truth, through reason and science ("the Enlightenment project"), has failed; our claims to truth and knowledge, whether through science or democracy or other ideologies, are merely culturally relative opinions, with economic and political sources. Our ideas (to adapt Marx) are a mere superstructure to our culture.

This way of thinking has taken root throughout Western culture. It began with the Romantic movement of the early nineteenth century, a protest against the rise of science, culminating most explicitly in the work of Nietzsche at the turn of the twentieth century. Many commentators think that it became associated with a certain nihilism, especially after the shock of the Great War of 1914–1918, which seemed to put the lie to the modernist notion of endless peace and prosperity. It seemed even more vindicated by the rise of Nazism in the very heart of the most modernist, scientific, rationalist Western nation—and the horror of the Holocaust, in which advanced technology was applied to evil purposes.

Postmodernism flourished in interwar France, especially under the influence of the philosopher Alexandre Kojeve, who mixed it with Marxism. The philosophy really took off in postwar France, spawning a generation of thinkers who fully formulated the postmodernist ideology, foremost among them Jean-Paul Sartre and Michel Foucault. The student revolts of 1968 are often seen as the practical flowering of the postmodernist rejection of liberal democracy and all its rationalist/scientific ideologies. The neoconservative reaction of the 1970s and 1980s followed, and the past few decades have been the setting of "culture wars" between postmodernism and conservatism among Western intellectuals.

THE POSTMODERNIST CRITIQUE IS, in great measure, a reaction to the science worship, called "positivism," of the nineteenth century. Yet the options are not the two extremes of postmodern nihilism or positivistic dogmatism. There are other perspectives, such as Karl Jaspers's pluralism (expanded in the Continental tradition of phenomenology) or William James's pragmatism (expanded later in the works of philosophers like W. V. O. Quine, Daniel Dennett, and others). There is a spectrum; but like all debates, the partisans at the extremes make the most noise.

The philosopher Daniel Dennett gave a remarkable lecture titled

"Postmodernism and Truth" in which he makes the point that post-modernist professors of literary theory can afford to be relativistic because they never get sued. Doctors don't have this luxury. If doctors can kill, and be sued, and held responsible for right and wrong action, then there are truths—hence postmodernism is false.

Postmodernist thinkers, like Foucault, have interpreted Nietzsche as arguing for a relativism of all morality, that ultimately power was the basis of all claims to the good. Contrary to these postmodernist misconceptions, one can say that Nietzsche was just arguing for a rational morality from the perspective of defining the good, as opposed to a morality (as in most of the Christian tradition) based on defining evil. Nietzsche was also trying to link morality to human psychology, making the point that different approaches to morality flowed from the state of humankind in different epochs of history. There is no unchanging essence to human nature, he claimed in agreement with Darwin, and thus our views of the moral would change based on the state of humankind in a certain time and place. This does not entail relativism: not all states of human nature are equally moral or praiseworthy; Nietzsche certainly had strong feelings on this point. Indeed, the postmodernist misappropriation of Nietzsche, just like the Nazi one, shows us that the problem is postmodernism itself, that those who claim to be diagnosing our ills are in fact their causes (a topic expanded in chapter 6).

Nietzsche had it right: Postmodernism is our disease today, but in case the German thinker and the academic phrase seem forbidding, we can turn to perhaps the most American of thinkers to confirm the problem; we can turn to Emerson (whom Nietzsche loved) and Thoreau.

WE ALL COMPLAIN ABOUT the dullness of life, Emerson taught; this is because we think that we ourselves, each one of us, matter. The melancholy of our leisure hours comes from this belief, he argued. I matter to myself, more than you, more than everyone, or almost everyone. If I matter so much, then it is a matter of great concern to me if I am in pain, or unhappy this moment, or unfulfilled. I matter; hence the world hurts.

I turn to diversions, seek wealth or position, all in response to the urge that I should satisfy my desire to matter.

I do not see that you matter too, indeed that many of you matter more than me, that any objective observer would fail to distinguish why I should matter more than you. But though I may think these thoughts, I matter to myself nonetheless, and I cannot help but wanting the world to bend to my wishes.

It is easy to counsel, as Emerson does, that the solution to this melancholy is to realize that I am a part of a larger whole; or to advise, as Martin Luther King does, that I cannot be who I want to be unless you can be who you want to be. This truth of interconnectedness—and it is a truth—satisfies reason at two in the afternoon but fails with desire at two in the morning.

And so we keep running about, trying to make our lives better, seeking prestige and recognition, sometimes succeeding, often failing, but even failing when we succeed, since the brief moments of fame are always followed by long hours of humdrum existence.

We keep going, trying to escape the ennui that gnaws behind in our lives of quiet desperation; Thoreau made the diagnosis and even proposed a special treatment. But two years in a wooden shed by a pond is not a practical option for most of us; and, even then, such therapy may work for any individual, but it fails societies, unless the dissolution of society be our aim.

Emerson and Thoreau are our diagnosticians, and they are indispensable since no treatment can work unless the diagnosis is true and valid. But for treatment of this diagnosis we must go elsewhere, and, before that, we must appreciate what the diagnosis means by deepening our appreciation of its hardened state, by learning what happens when mild melancholy becomes deep depression, by turning to profound pathology to better comprehend the prosaic pain of our daily lives.

CHAPTER 2

The Varieties of Depressive Experience

THERE IS A MEDICAL syndrome of childhood, a genetic disease, in which the child does not develop pain receptors in the skin. Called *congenital anesthesia*, this disease involves genetic mutations in sodium channels in the dorsal roots of the spinal cord such that pain fibers do not function. The syndrome is dangerous, because as children grow, they bang their limbs in various places, but they don't recoil with pain, and thus excessive damage occurs to the skin without their realizing it. Infections follow, and inevitably, chronic sores and deep tissue damage leads to the loss of limbs, severe infection throughout the body, and death.

We experience pain so that we may live; without pain, we die. This is the case with physical pain in the body, and it is the case with mental pain in the brain. There is, perhaps, a key functional role for depression in human existence. When we become depressed, it is a sign that we are at a dead end; perhaps our judgments were wrong about something or someone, and we should change course. Depression, like pain, has a meaning. Our job is not simply to eradicate it but also to find out what it means.

DEPRESSION AS A CLINICAL problem, an illness, something that leads to psychological or medical attention, is not the same thing as sadness. One is sad, to be sure, but there is much more. Physical symptoms predominate: sleep is disturbed, the body is tired, the will is absent to do simple things, like shower and shave and dress. Sometimes, one hardly moves out of the bed, or movements become sluggish, as if air itself had become viscous. Memory might begin to fail, focusing on

---

We experience pain so that we may live; without pain, we die

---

tasks would be difficult, one could begin to feel dumb. Self-accusations would follow; I must be to blame to feel so horrible, or I brought my problems on myself; I should have been better, smarter, stronger. Suicide seems reasonable: all is pain; there may only seem one way out.

This is clinical depression; it is a lot more than feeling sad, but it grows out of a deep and painful sadness, which starts at the core of one's soul, radiates out to one's body, and then engulfs one's entire being.

It becomes a chokehold, this depression, enveloping the self from the inside out and not letting go for weeks, months, sometimes even a year or more. This too marks sickness from sadness; the healthy are sad for days, the sick are depressed for weeks, the melancholic are immobilized for months. The process has a dark beginning and a dark end.

This description is a distillation of reality; no single depression has all these features, most depressions have some. Depressive experiences come in many shapes, not only in the way they are experienced but also in how they came to happen in the first place.

THERE ARE MANY DEPRESSIVE varieties to be explored. For some people, clinical depression is always there, to a greater or lesser degree, and it never goes away. Under the stresses of life, the constant low-level depression becomes worse, if only for a few weeks or a few months; it is like a constant dull headache that suddenly becomes sharp now and again. Someone dies; I have a tough meeting with my boss; a bus almost hits me; a bully bothers my child in school. These stresses happen to all of us: we don't develop clinical depression as a result. But some people, who constantly have the dull headache of low-level depression, will sink into deep depressive funks after the meeting with the boss and not come out until months later, at which time they go back to their usual life of the dull headache—a baseline mild depression. We used to have a name for this condition, no longer used in psychiatry today: "neurotic depression." Usually the baseline depression is admixed with some anxiety symptoms, a general worrywart attitude, a pessimism, and a fear about life. Hence the term "neurotic." I think the old term—now discarded for the fancier terms "dysthymia" and "generalized anxiety disorder"—was more true to reality. There is a depression there, but it is neurotic and chronic.

Some people have a different kind of depression: Sometimes they are deeply sick, severely depressed, suicidal, and nonfunctional; these black depths last months and months but rarely longer than a year. When not deeply melancholic, these persons are well (or near-well, with a slight sadness, called "dysthymic"). They are not a little depressed, or generally anxious; they are well, like you and me and that 90 percent of the population that never experiences clinical depression of any kind. In other words, they have depressive episodes, which come and go, and they have periods when they are completely (or near-completely) healthy. This is episodic depression, and it either happens alone (called "unipolar") or with manic periods (called "bipolar").

There is a third group: Some people are fully healthy, without a symptom of depression, and have a severe depressive episode, and then never have another one. About one-third of persons who have a severe depressive episode are in this category: they have a single episode their entire lives.

A fourth group is fully healthy until they have a stroke, or a heart attack, or develop cancer, and then for the first, and last, time in their lives they have a depressive episode. If the medical illness is cured, they never have another depression.

All four of these varieties of depression are currently given the same label in modern psychiatry: "major depressive disorder," known by its initials, MDD. Some of their differences may be signaled by adding other labels (e.g., "major depressive disorder with the comorbidity of generalized anxiety disorder"), but the MDD label is the diagnosis.

There is little doubt we have a spectrum here: it ranges from neurotic low-level depressive and anxiety symptoms that are chronic to a single depressive episode (with or without a medical cause) to recurrent depressive episodes.

It has become de rigueur to state that depression is a disease. I would say the opposite: most depression is not a disease. The part of it that is recurrent and episodic, or due to a specific medical cause, is disease. But the part that is not episodic, that is chronic and admixed with anxiety, becomes indistinguishable from personality; though it seems similar to the disease of recurrent severe depression, it does not have similar biological causes, nor does it derive similar benefit from biological treatments.

LET ME USE SHORTHAND: I will call recurrent severe depression "Depression disease"; I will call neurotic and single episode depression "Depression nondisease." We can conceive of the spectrum of clinical depression as having causes that are either biological, environmental, or a mix. While the mix of the two is common, it is relevant that sometimes depression is purely biological and sometimes purely environmental. Let me provide some admittedly extreme examples to show how this could be. Let us assume in these examples, as happens in real life, that the duration of depressive episodes is determined naturally, that it begins and ends on its own, and that no treatment is given. Someone may have had ten recurrent episodes of severe depression, each lasting six months, with six months of completely normal mood in between each episode. That person may have a family history of severe depression and suicides for three generations. Each episode in that person occurs spontaneously, untriggered by any life stressors. This is a purely biological depression—definitely Depression disease.

Someone else may never have had a symptom of depression for fifty years, then experience a divorce, have a clinical depression for three months, and then never experience a symptom of depression for another forty years in a long life that is followed to the end. This is definitely a purely environmental cause—Depression nondisease.

Now we come to the mix—those whose depressive periods involve a combination of genetic or biological and environmental factors. Some persons in the family may have depression, but most don't; most episodes are associated with apparently related life events; and the episodes are recurrent, not occurring just once. Periods of fully normal mood also occur between episodes, though sometimes low-level depressive symptoms persist between episodes. This scenario is clinically more common, at least in typical psychiatric practice settings, than the highly biological or highly environmental types of depression described above. Genetic studies of twins also show that an almost equal mix of genetic and environmental factors seem to be involved with such cases of MDD.

This mix of biology and environment needs to be examined, though, like the recipe of an entree: What are its ingredients?

LET'S START WITH THE environment part, and to do so, we'll go back to that old sage, Aristotle, and take some ideas about causes from him (what follows is not solely what Aristotle said, but what I would derive from his ideas, adding my own views, as relevant to understanding depression). Aristotle's key insight was that if we want to understand what causes what, we have to appreciate that there are different types of causes. In my interpretation of how these ideas are relevant to depression today, I think we can at least clarify two basic classes of causes: those that reflect an underlying susceptibility to depression and those that trigger, or immediately precede, a period of depression. Let's call the former the "first cause" and the latter the "efficient cause." (For Aristotle, the first cause was the initial efficient cause that set everything else in motion. Though this idea has mostly been discussed in relation to proving God's existence—what Aristotle called the Unmoved Mover—it is relevant to understanding diseases like depression.) The first cause is the initial biological susceptibility to depression; without it, later efficient causes would have no effect. One of the greatest errors in understanding depression is to mistake first and efficient causes, or susceptibility and triggers.

The first cause in depression is genetics and early life environment; without these unchanging susceptibilities, later efficient causes could never produce a clinical depressive episode. The efficient causes are the immediate life events that trigger a clinical depression *at that time*—the divorce, the job loss, or the death that precedes *this* episode of depression. The first cause is *necessary* for later depression though not *sufficient*; it usually is not enough to lead to the actual depressive episodes of adult life. The efficient causes are not *necessary*—depression can occur without them, and the same life events occur without depression in other people, and even in the same person they do not invariably produce depression—but they sometimes are *sufficient*: in some persons they can lead to depression whenever they occur.

So first causes are necessary but usually not sufficient; efficient causes are often sufficient but not necessary. One usually needs both, and neither alone is *the* cause of depression.

A common mistake is to see the efficient cause as *the* cause of a depressive episode. This is a commonsense mistake, one that flows logically from our usual daily judgments, and one that is often repeated by mental health clinicians. The efficient cause often seems to be the sole cause because of the temporal relation: the efficient cause happens, then the depression happens; one would seem to cause the other; first *x*, then *y*, means that *x* causes *y*. In daily living, this is common sense. But in the case of psychiatric problems like clinical depression, common sense fails. If common sense would have clarified matters, then patients would not need to come to clinicians; they would have had their problems handled by their family or friends, by the standard application of commonsense thinking. Mental health clinicians should be biased *against* common sense, because anything that comes their way has already failed to respond to it.

Besides this logical rationale for why efficient causes should be deemphasized, there is a strong biological rationale, based on split-brain studies in neurology. These studies are so important for the understanding of how we think that we could use them as a basis for all that we do in psychiatry: let's call it *split-brain psychiatry*.

IN SOME EPILEPSIES, WHERE seizures don't respond well to medications, surgery is sometimes used as a treatment: the fibers connecting the right and left hemisphere (called the *corpus callosum*) are cut. After corpus callosotomy, seizures that begin on one side of the brain don't travel to the other side, and full-blown convulsions are thus prevented.

This kind of surgery began a few decades ago, and, in the intervening time, researchers have observed an important thing about these patients: living with two halves of a brain no longer communicating with each other, it is as if they have two brains, not one. Not much is noticeable in terms of personality or behavior; interacting on the street or in stores, one cannot tell someone with a split brain, after corpus callosotomy, apart from the rest of us. With neuropsychological tests, however, important abnormalities emerge.

The right hemisphere of the brain controls the left visual field; the left hemisphere controls the right visual field. In all right-handed persons, language is fully controlled by the left hemisphere. (In left-handed persons, language is partly controlled by both hemispheres.) Thus, in right-handed patients after split-brain surgery, the split between language and vision can be tested. If an image is shown to the right hemisphere (in the left visual field), say, of a woman talking on a phone, the experimenter who asks the patient, "What do you see?" will get an answer, a wrong answer, but an answer nonetheless: "I see a friend" the person might say. What is the friend doing? "Cooking dinner." Then with a phone nearby, the experimenter can ask the subject, "Show me what you saw." The person will pick up the phone, with her left hand.

The split-brain epilepsy patient "knows" what is seen by the right hemisphere, but she cannot speak it. What is most interesting is that she does not say, "I don't know," or "I am unsure," or some such. Sometimes the researcher says: Now remember, you have had split-brain surgery for your seizures; keep that in mind when you answer my questions. Still, patients rarely say that they don't know what they saw, or why they feel as they do about what they saw. They rarely admit ignorance; they usually make something up. That is the way our brains operate: Our brains are rationalizing machines; we are designed, by God or evolution, to come up with plausible explanations for what we experience. *We don't say we don't know.*

That is the basic axiom upon which one can build a scientific edifice of split-brain psychiatry.

IT SEEMS, WHEN WE are depressed, that something happened just beforehand, so it must have *caused* us to become depressed. First *x* happens, then *y*; so *x* must *cause* *y*. Long ago the philosopher David Hume noted this fact: we tend to attribute causation to the *constant conjunction* of events. First *x*, then *y*; first *x*, then *y*; first *x*, then *y*; when these two events follow one upon the other, over and over again, we conclude practically that *x* causes *y*. This makes sense, at some level, but it isn't proof. Even after a million times of *y* following *x*, it could be that *x* might occur without *y* following it one time. There is no guarantee that *x* absolutely leads to *y*. This was Hume's observation, to use philosophical language, that we infer causation based on induction of observations; such induction is not infallible, only probabilistic, Hume claimed.

Call it *Hume's fallacy*—the notion that an association of events is enough to infer causation. This fallacy is stronger when there might be a conjunction, but not a *constant* conjunction. So I got depressed after my girlfriend left me; then I got depressed after the stock market fell; then I got depressed after George W. Bush was elected president. I can attribute each depression to what happened around that time, to Aristotle's efficient cause, using the reasoning that Hume identified as part of human nature. But I would be wrong, partly because each depression is associated with a *different* event (not a constant conjunction with the same event), and partly because my split brain is wired so that I come up with some kind of explanation or another.

This discussion becomes relevant to much of the debate about the official psychiatric diagnostic system, the *Diagnostic and Statistical Manual of Mental Disorders*, or *DSM* (see chapter 9). Some have criticized a proposal for the fifth edition to remove an exclusion criterion for grief in relation to depression. In other words, depression would be diagnosed even in the setting of grief after someone's death. These critics argue that there should be a separate diagnostic category of depression that is "caused by" or "understandable" given certain psychosocial events or stressors.

These are facile assumptions: Something bad happens, *therefore* I'm depressed. Where does that *therefore* come from? It comes from our split brains, our commonsense reliance on Hume's fallacy, and it's often wrong.

THIS IS NOT to say that efficient causes are not causes, but to say that they are not the sole causes. All those life stressors *trigger*, but aren't the sole cause of, those episodes.

Aristotle's first cause looms behind. Why is it that I had a major depressive episode when Bush got elected, and you, equally fervently a Democrat, didn't? Why is it that I had a major depressive episode when my girlfriend left me, and you, equally enamored by your sweetheart, didn't?

There is something about my inherent susceptibility to getting a severe depression, with these same life stressors, that you don't have. My first cause is there; yours is not.

In biological language, we often speak of a mixture of genetics and environment as being the etiologies—causes—of depression. Genetics and early life environment can be seen as a first cause, the underlying susceptibility to getting depressed later; and later environmental stresses are the efficient causes, the triggers of exactly when and how one gets depressed.

The biological susceptibility, the first cause, is necessary but usually not sufficient to cause depression. The adult environmental triggers, the efficient causes, are often sufficient but not necessary.

A PRIME FEATURE OF the genetics of depression, rarely emphasized, is that it proves Freud wrong. Genetic studies on twins can differentiate between the input of genes and environment, because identical twins share all their genes, and fraternal twins only half, while all will share similar family environment. Mathematical equations can model the likely risks of illness due to genes, which come in two varieties, mendelian and additive. Mendelian genes add large amounts of risk, 50 percent likelihood if they are dominant and 25 percent likelihood if they are recessive. Additive genes each add a small amount of risk, but no single gene adds much risk. The effects of additive genes are less than 25 percent risk (e.g., 10 percent or less for any single gene). Given the mathematical observation of depression prevalence in twins, it is clear that the genetic risk for depression is additive—many genes are needed, each with a small contribution to risk (a nonmendelian process).

The mathematical models also tell us how environment influences depression; they divide environment into two varieties: shared and unshared. Shared environment is what twins experience the same way, namely family and culture. Specific, or unshared, environment is what they experience differently, such as different random experiences in life or different peer groups. Possibly, children who are not twins will have different family experiences due to differing birth order (older children tend to be treated different from younger children).

It turns out that the underlying susceptibility for depression, its first cause, involves additive genes and specific environment. There are no mendelian genes—no single genes—that cause the illness more or less by themselves. And there are few shared environmental risks: the family, culture, society are not major causes of depression.

So, these twin studies prove Freud wrong: it doesn't matter how the child feels toward his mother or her father; the Oedipus complex (which Freud saw as a universal stage of childhood development) is irrelevant; most of the vagaries of child-parent relationships are unimportant. None of those family relations, the core of the inner psychological world of psychoanalysis, have any major causative role for depression.

Other aspects of specific environment may be relevant, but exactly what they are remains to be proven. One possible feature could be childhood trauma, often sexual in nature; if severe trauma occurs in some children but not all it could conceivably be a risk factor. Parental loss, the death of a parent, is also a specific event that is a risk factor for later depression. Family life may still be relevant to the extent that children are treated differently; sibling order sometimes influences the environment for one child in a different way from another. Peer relationships are an important potential specific environmental influence that might be related to depression.

When we think of environment, we can still think of salient social factors, but we need to remember that they need to be specific to the individual, not shared among children, to match up with the twin studies.

Often it is assumed that the environment must inherently involve social factors. Yet environment can still reflect biology; we have a biological environment: bacteria and viruses buzz around us. Some research suggests that a major risk factor for mental illnesses, including severe depression and bipolar disorder, is infection during pregnancy. Intrauterine infection in the second trimester in particular may be a risk factor for later psychiatric illness. Psychiatric conditions are more common in children born during influenza epidemics.

So the combination of additive genes and specific environment need not translate into a combination of biology and psychosocial factors; it could be wholly biological on both sides or at least mostly so.

Another way this could all work, again with a primacy for biology, would be in what is called "gene by environment interaction." The mathematical modeling of twins was based on the assumption that one could simply add up the effects of genes and specific environment to explain the frequency of depression. The models assumed that genes and environment do not interact, such that, if you have certain genes, you are no more likely to have certain environments or the reverse. But other studies indicate that it is highly likely that such interaction occurs. So it appears that if a child's genetics predispose her to behave in a certain way, she will elicit a certain reaction in her environment, different from the environmental experience of another child whose genetics predispose him to behave in another way. So there may be a synergistic effect: to oversimplify, if your genes are "bad" (psychologically, let's say, they make you more likely to be depressed), then your environment is more likely to be "bad" (your depressive behavior will elicit negative feedback from others, which will make you more depressed). And vice versa. This is gene and environment interaction, and it could be another reason why the environmental risks are specific to the individual, perhaps because that person's specific genetic makeup is likely to elicit those environmental risks.

CULTURE, THE LARGER SHARED environment, has no major role in the etiology of the disease of depression, as a first cause, based on the twin studies. But culture may have a role in the *expression* of depression, especially in its nondisease forms.

Few are depressed in Taiwan; every fifth person is depressed in Paris. In a large international epidemiological study, well-trained researchers went out, knocked on doors, interviewed people, and applied *DSM-IV* (the fourth revision of the *DSM*) criteria for psychiatric disorders. Only 1 percent of the population in Taiwan can be diagnosed with MDD, that is having had a major depressive episode at some point in life; almost 20 percent of the population in Paris meet that definition. It's about 1 percent in Iran, about 5 percent in the United States, 10 percent in Canada. Why all this fluctuation?

In contrast, the prevalence of schizophrenia and bipolar disorder, in those same studies, is about 1 percent no matter which country is examined.

What's different about depression? One can only repeat: Depression (unlike bipolar disorder and schizophrenia) is not a disease. At least not depression when defined as MDD, using the *DSM-IV* definition. It is a mixture of some presentations that are disease (recurrent episodic major depressive episodes, as described above) and some that are not (neurotic depression, as described above). The neurotic depression presentation in Paris is expressed psychologically in terms of mood and interest and apathy; in Taipei, or Tehran, or Shanghai, it is expressed as headache, back pain, physical exhaustion, and a myriad of somatic symptoms that keep doctors busy and wealthy, tending somatically to somatic symptoms that have no somatic cause. (*Dat Galenus opes*: Galen—medicine—gives wealth, goes the old saying.)

If culture is relevant to depression, it is in showing what is not disease and in reminding us that neurotic depressive symptoms, the nondisease form, vary markedly in how they are expressed from culture to culture.

THE WRITER H. L. MENCKEN once commented that Puritanism is the haunting fear that someone, somewhere may be happy. At some level, our American culture, haunted by its Pilgrim past, accepts a psychopharmacological Calvinism, the notion that, if pills make you feel good, then they must be bad. We are also a hedonistic society, happily living in the age of Prozac, where we defend taking pills to make you smarter, or sharper, or more productive, or just plain happier. I have to take care of me, and what matters is what makes me feel better. Advertisers know that our desires can be manufactured: what makes me feel better is not something that I decide, by myself, but rather something I am convinced to believe by what I see on television advertisements, magazine pictures, and Times Square billboards. So I feel I need these pills because I have been led to believe, by those pharmaceutical marketers, that I need these pills.

So how do I know what's right? Is my rejection of pills an unconscious Calvinism, rationally indefensible and ultimately based on a cultural theology? Is my acceptance of pills an unconscious hedonism, only superficially my own but really a cultural artifact of Madison Avenue puppeteers?

If some depression is disease, and needs medications, but other kinds of depression are not disease and may not need or benefit from medications, we are left with a dilemma. Our acceptance or rejection of antidepressants cannot occur in a cultural vacuum; culturally, we

---

What makes me feel better is not something that I decide, by myself, but rather something I am convinced to believe by what I see on television advertisements, magazine pictures, and Times Square billboards

---

are pulled in both directions, excessive caution versus overweening acceptance of antidepressants (more on this in chapter 4).

IT WOULD SEEM THAT the key feature of depression as a disease is depression itself. Most books about depression go into detail about specific symptoms of depression: typical features (decreased sleep and decreased appetite), atypical features (increased sleep and increased appetite), melancholic features (early morning awakening, marked lack of feeling), psychotic features (presence of delusions or hallucinations), and so on.

My view is that none of this matters much.

Instead, the key to understanding the disease of depression is not the depression itself, but the coming and going of it; not the actual episode of depression and its features, but the mere existence of depression, and how frequently it comes and goes; in a word, not the episode itself, but the fact of recurrence of episodes.

Recurrence, not the symptoms of depressive episodes themselves, is the hallmark of the disease of depression. This was the view of that great Germanic psychiatrist (not Freud) who laid the foundations of twentieth-century psychiatric diagnosis: Emil Kraepelin. Kraepelin saw mental illness as divided into two categories: dementia praecox (literally, "precocious dementia," later called schizophrenia) dealt with disordered thinking and manic-depressive insanity dealt with moods. This was referred to as the Kraepelinian dichotomy.

While many view today's diagnostic manual as neo-Kraepelinian, it is only partly so. Versions since 1980 (*DSM-III* and on) have labeled most mood conditions as variations on depression: a very broad major depressive disorder (MDD) category, with numerous variants (dysthymia, adjustment disorder with depressed mood, secondary mood disorder). Kraepelin cared not for depression, seeing most depressive conditions as part of his larger category of manic-depressive insanity (MDI). Many assume that MDI is now translated as bipolar disorder, but in fact Kraepelin's MDI would correspond to today's bipolar disorder *plus MDD*. For Kraepelin, the key feature of MDI was *recurrence* of *any kind* of mood episodes, depression *or* (not *and*) mania. Thus, ten depressive episodes was MDI; ten manic episodes was also MDI. What matters is the number of episodes, not the kind of mood state.

He recognized that some people only have a single episode of depression. This nonrecurrent depression he limited to the use of the diagnosis of "melancholia." If melancholia was recurrent, it was seen as MDI.

Manic-depressive insanity, a recurrent illness, was a "disease process." Melancholia, a nonepisodic condition, wasn't a disease but was rather a "clinical picture," much like backache and muscle soreness is a clinical picture.

Clinical pictures, when investigated, sometimes represent disease processes (think: fever, chills, and headache due to meningitis), and sometimes they don't (think: the common headache of unknown cause). In the former case they *always* require medical treatment (intravenous antibiotics are needed or else one dies); in the latter case they sometimes, perhaps frequently, don't (take two aspirin and call me in the morning).

In today's psychiatry, where all MDD is viewed as biological illness, and the distinction between recurrence and nonrecurrence is ignored, we are taking two antidepressants tonight, and the next day, and the next day, forever. We have forgotten the Hippocratic wisdom of the great physician Lewis Thomas: "The great secret, known to internists and learned very early in marriage by their wives, but still hidden from the general public, is that most things get better by themselves. Most things in fact are better by the morning."

USUALLY DEPRESSION IS SEEN as harmful. The prevailing theory about it is that depression distorts our perception of reality, it makes our thoughts abnormally negative, and we see the world darkly and unjustly. This cognitive distortion model of depression, the basis for the popular cognitive-behavioral therapy (CBT), is not unchallenged. Another model argues the exact opposite: depression leads to enhanced contact with reality, perhaps to the detriment of the depressed.

In classic experiments, psychologists gave depression rating scales to college students and then experimental tests where the students were asked to do things. The students had control over how the tests would go; if they did one thing, they could expect a certain result, and if they did another thing, another result, and so on. At some point, though, without telling the students, the researchers rigged the test so that it would respond randomly to the students; student control over what would happen next was removed. Then the magic of this research: some students could tell that they had less control, but others persisted in thinking they were in control. Those who realized what had happened, dubbed the more "realistic" students, also had higher scores on depression symptoms; those who persisted in feeling they were in control though they were not, the less realistic students,

---

A little depression—not too much—makes you more realistic

---

had low or no depressive symptoms at all. A little depression—not too much—makes you more realistic. No depression—none at all, being fully mentally healthy—makes you less realistic. Illusion is part of being sane, but it comes at a cost.

I could tell a story about how in fact, in the course of regular human affairs, a little illusion is good. If I didn't think this book was somewhat better than it really is likely to be, I wouldn't spend all this effort in writing it. If you didn't think your life is more worthwhile than an objective Martian, watching from outer space, might conclude, you wouldn't work hard and pay the bills and take the family out to dinner. I am often struck by all the effort that parents put into their children's education. We stress over preschool, and elementary school, and beyond; we pay high bills for private schools, and we analyze public schools carefully; we care to have the best teachers and we push our kids for the best grades; we hope they'll get into Ivy League schools—and then? Is it not simply a realistic fact, a statistical one, that most of our children, even if they get the best training and go to their Ivy League school of choice, will end up as one of many accountants, and lawyers, and bureaucrats, and doctors (nothing against any of these professions)? But they won't be much greater, if any, than we are, or than our parents were; they likely won't be presidents of the United States, or presidents of companies, or even make it to city hall. And yet we think they will; that's the bit of self-illusion that we all have, we nondepressed happy human beings.

The depressive realism hypothesis is this: Depressed persons are not depressed because they distort reality; they are depressed because they see reality more clearly than we nondepressed people do.

Which raises the question: Is there something abnormal about being happy?

CHAPTER 3

Abnormal Happiness

THERE IS SUCH A THING as abnormal happiness. Few write books about it, though, because we tend to see happiness as a purely positive goal, devoutly to be wished. We assume—and a whole recent psychological genre of "happiness studies" has not challenged this assumption—that happiness is inherently good; hence the natural inclination to think of despair and depression as inherently bad. Once we allow for the insight that not all depression is hurtful, then we might be prepared for the judgment that not all happiness is desirable.

The psychiatric term for abnormal happiness is *mania*. Here mood is classically elated, sometimes giddy, often alternating with anger. Time is sped up. One doesn't need to sleep much; everything is going twice as fast. Four hours can do it. While the rest of the world is sleeping, one's energy is running like it's 11 a.m. on a Wednesday: why not clean the entire house at 3 a.m.? Things need to get done, even if they don't. Redecorate the house; do it again; buy a third car. Work two hours longer daily: the boss loves it. One's thoughts pour forth; the brain seems to be much faster than the mouth. Trying to keep up with those rapid thoughts, one speaks quickly, interrupting others, running a conversation from only one end. Friends and coworkers get annoyed; they can't get a word in edgewise. This may produce more irritability; why can't everyone else get up to speed? "Mania is extremity for one's friends," Robert Lowell remarked, "depression for oneself." Sex becomes even more appealing; one's spouse may like it, or might tire of it. The urge is so strong that one might look to satisfy it elsewhere; affairs are common; divorce is the rule; HIV rates are high. Self-esteem rises; sometimes, it

---

"Mania is extremity for one's friends," Robert Lowell remarked, "depression for oneself"

---

leads to great successes, where one's skills were up to the task; too frequently, it leads to equally grand failures, where circumstances overwhelm one. But there is no past; there is hardly today; only the future counts, and, there, anything is possible. Decisions become easy to make; no guilt, no doubt. *Just do it.* The trouble is not in starting things but in ending them; so much to do, so little time, it's easy to get distracted.

Ultimately, bad decisions might get made; too impulsive, these bad decisions stereotypically fall into four categories: sexual indiscretions, spending sprees, reckless driving, and impulsive traveling. The car becomes a dangerous extension of one's powerful self; accidents, poor driving records, and lethal risks are not uncommon. Traveling is a preferred mode of life: it seems decisive, and things must be better somewhere else. Living in numerous places in a year is typical. Or simply visiting someplace with no plans seems reasonable. Divorce, debt, sexually transmitted diseases, occupational instability—mania is the perfect antidote to the cherished simple goals of most persons: a family, a home, a job, a stable life. In depression, one takes one's life; in mania, one ruins one's life. In manic-depressive illness, one suffers from both tragic risks.

"NORMAL" HAPPINESS TENDS to be seen as contextual: If I win the lottery, I'm happy. Good things happen, one feels happy. Psychiatrists call this *normal mood reactivity*: the ability to react normally to good or bad news with happier or sadder mood, respectively.

The problem with this definition, though it is not in itself false, is that abnormal happiness and abnormal depression also often, in fact usually, have a context. This is because of the split-brain nature of our minds: we provide rationalized contexts for everything we feel. But the feeling comes first, the rationalization comes later. The feeling is always right, the rationalization often wrong.

In the old days, before the split-brain studies, moods were distinguished based on these supposed causes. Depression was "reactive," caused by some painful experience in the environment, and thus not biological; or it was "endogenous," occurring without any environmental cause, and thus biological. We now know this is untrue: many depressive periods that are part of diseases like manic-depressive illness are triggered, though not caused, by some life event. (The difference between a trigger and a cause is important, as described in chapter 2.)

Although this concept has long been debated in relation to depression, it has not been discussed in relation to happiness. Implicitly, we've tended to use this same commonsense, though mistaken, notion: If someone is happy "because" x and y happened, then that happiness is normal. Only if nothing in the world has happened, and someone is inexplicably happy, do we consider that he or she might be manic.

A GOOD EXAMPLE of this kind of assumption is found in a recent study of German psychologists, to whom researchers gave two vignettes of a person with severe depression and another person with mania. The cases were set up so as to clearly meet *DSM-IV* definitions of a major depressive episode and a manic episode. The psychologists were asked to diagnose the cases as major depression, mania, or neither. Ninety-five percent correctly diagnosed the case of *DSM-IV* defined major depression; only 38 percent diagnosed the case of mania correctly (53 percent saw it as depression!). The researchers put in a wrinkle: half of the vignettes for the case of mania stated that the male in the case (who had happy mood, decreased need for sleep, increased activity level, increased talkativeness, and impulsive behavior) had just started a new relationship with a girlfriend; the other half of the vignettes for the case of mania said nothing about any external trigger for the symptoms. In the girlfriend case, the correct diagnosis of mania dropped to 23 percent; in the non-girlfriend case, it rose to 60 percent.

Girlfriends, especially new ones, tend to make men happy, but not manic—not, at least, without a strong biological susceptibility to bipolar disorder.

Having a girlfriend or not is irrelevant to determining whether a person is experiencing a manic episode; yet most of us think this way naturally, as with the psychologists in that study. This is common sense but it's wrong. Science is about learning when and why to reject common sense. Split-brain psychiatry teaches us that common sense is frequently erroneous and definitely shouldn't be presumed regularly veracious.

ONE CAN'T EASILY DEFINE normal happiness, certainly not from its relation to external life events.

Perhaps we should instead seek to define abnormal varieties of happiness. (An excellent source for this material is a recently translated early twentieth-century dissertation by the German psychiatrist William Mayer-Gross, under the supervision of the great philosopher and psychiatrist Karl Jaspers. Mayer-Gross, who later emigrated to the United Kingdom and had a major influence on twentieth-century British psychiatry, pulled together fascinating nineteenth-century sources, including the work of the philosopher William James and others.) One approach would be to view abnormal happiness as occurring when the emotion totally takes over one's mind: all of one's thoughts and feelings are imbued with happiness. In contrast, normal happiness might be partial: we are happy about this or that, but not in a general or absolute sense about everything. James called the absolute experience of happiness "ecstasy" and the psychologist Kay Jamison refers to it as "exuberance." To provide examples, James turns to the experience of patients with mania (including himself) and the rapturous experiences of religious mystics. Here is an example that James reported from the experience of a mystic:

> Last night was the sweetest night I ever had in my life. I never before, for so long a time together, enjoyed so much of the light and rest and sweetness of heaven in my soul, but without the least agitation of body during

the whole time. . . . all night I continued in a constant, clear, and lively sense of the heavenly sweetness of Christ's excellent love, of his nearness to me, and of my dearness to him; with an inexpressibly sweet calmness of soul. . . . I seemed to myself to perceive a glow of divine love down from the heart of Christ in heaven into my heart in a constant stream, like a stream or pencil of sweet light. . . . I appeared to myself to float or swim, in these bright, sweet beams, like the moats swimming in the beams of the sun. . . . It was pleasure, without the least sting, or any interruption. It was sweetness which my soul was lost in; it seemed to be all that my feeble frame could sustain.

It could be that this kind of complete mind-filling euphoria is behind the mystical experience of union with the outside world. Everything seems the same as me, and I seem a part of everything around me, because the parts of me have disappeared inside this mind-saturating experience of ecstasy. The self dissolves in the outside world.

ANOTHER KIND OF ABNORMAL happiness is not characterized, as is ecstasy, by a complete overtaking of the mind. This happiness is abnormal not because it is absolute but because it isn't real. We aren't realistically happy because good things are going on around us; we are just happy inside our minds, and then we project that happiness onto the outside world. Our happiness doesn't extend over the whole world, the abstract universe, God, but rather in concrete objects, engendering a sense of jubilation that pushes one to express it, either in words or actions. Here is a mid-nineteenth-century description:

I was lifted up by soft clouds, it was as if with every passing minute my mind was freed from its fetters, and inexpressible delight and gratitude entered my heart. . . . A wholly new, celestial life began within me. . . . My ideas surged forward so that I now contradicted what I had enthusiastically proclaimed just an hour before. But I was indescribably cheerful and seemed transfigured. . . . I was in an enviable state at the time, such as I had always wished for. In truth, I experienced a foretaste of heaven within my soul. . . . The world and humanity smiled at me, I longed for action so that I could start life anew. . . . My voice suddenly became light and clear,

I sang all the time. . . . every face appeared to me unrecognizably more beautiful. . . . I wanted to make the whole world happy through my own self-sacrifice and to resolve all conflicts.

Emotions sublimes, the French psychologist Pierre Janet called it, combined with a push to action. This experience, which is typical of a manic episode, is so pleasurable that it contradicts our association of disease with suffering. Writes one person with the condition:

"I do not know why I use the term illness, because subjectively I have never felt better. Sometimes I thought my vigour and productivity had doubled; it seemed to me that I knew and understood everything; my imagination gave me endless joy."

Nor is this heightened potency merely emotional; it is also physical, especially sexual: one's muscles feel stronger, Janet wrote; one's sexual drive is heightened, libido surges, sex is pleasurable, frequent, and varied in its fulfillment.

A pleasurable disease, this mania.

YET AS PLEASURE IS closely allied to pain, so is this extreme happiness easily tipped over into anger and dysphoria. If after all, I am so intelligent, why doesn't the rest of the world recognize it as so? I should be able to reach the president; he needs to hear from me, since I know more than all others around him. The converse of my intelligence can be reflected in the unknowing lack of recognition by others, in the idiocy of those around me. When my pleasure collides with the world's reality, love quickly turns to hate and joy to rage.

It's for this reason that most manic episodes involve anger and not just pure euphoria. This is one reason why manic episodes are not unalloyed experiences of rapture. One of my patients wanted too much sex when he became manic; his girlfriend gave him some, but she had her limits. Then he would get mad and even physically threatening to her. Needless to say, the relationship didn't last.

Then, there is the unavoidable psychological law of gravity that whoever is granted access to that kind of high must at some point come down, and fast. The price of mania is depression.

Next, the worst, unfortunately common, outcome: the energy and power of mania, and the moods and climate of depression, mixed together. As one of my patients' wives put it of her husband with bipolar disorder: "In our house, he was like the weather, completely unpredictable. One moment, he'd be nice, the next he'd bite your head off. You can't live with someone like that."

There are many varieties of abnormal types of happiness, and they are not all happy ones.

Yet, in our postmodern culture, we don't think deeply about happiness; we even think it might be found in a capsule.

CHAPTER 4

The Age of Prozac

TOWARD THE END OF the 1980s, the age of Aquarius gave way to the age of Prozac, as many Americans came to seek enlightenment, or some measure of happiness, through psychiatric medications, particularly a new generation of antidepressants with few side effects, the first of which was Prozac. Peter Kramer documented the change in *Listening to Prozac*. He argued there that Prozac, and by extension other new antidepressants, do more than treat severe clinical depression. Rather, in persons who had some depressive symptoms, but not full severe depressive episodes, Prozac seemed to provide new insights into life and free people up from inhibitions and limitations of personality. What Kramer was suggesting, which was revolutionary, was that psychopharmacology not only was needed for severe psychiatric illnesses but also could help with daily problems of living that previously were occasions for seeking psychotherapy. Patients didn't go from being sick to being normal; they went from being normal to being "better than well."

I remember seeing people like those Kramer described. I once treated a timid young woman; nervously, and at odd intervals, she sucked at her water bottle, as if it could provide the comfort that the rest of the world denied her. She was slightly chubby, pale, and had an innocence to her; she looked like she came from a place where the air was pure and the terrain expansive, and she did. North Dakota, however, was too boring. So she left home at 18 and came to Boston; she worked as a nanny, spent money on clothes rather than school, and had been seeking an end to her boredom ever since. "I'm disconnected from everyone else," she complained—her boyfriend and the forty girls who lived with her in a rooming house notwithstanding. As far as she was concerned, she lived alone in a crowd of strangers. So when she saw a friend taking Prozac, she decided to try it. One a day for a month; she didn't need a doctor to tell her how to do it. And it worked. "How did Prozac affect you?" I asked. "It was like putting on glasses for the first time," she replied. "Everything suddenly became clear." But without a doctor, her friend's supply ran out, and she sunk down again into her pure innocent disconnected world.

Along with prescribing medications, Kramer also practiced psychotherapy; indeed his first book was about couples' relationships. What struck him was that many individuals did not make progress in psychotherapy, but, with a brief period on Prozac, they achieved many of the changes in their personality styles that had been resistant to longer periods of intensive psychotherapy.

So the question he raised was a deep one: Beyond treating the illness of depression, do the new antidepressants provide a means to make non-depressed people happy? Is Prozac the solution to the puzzle of happiness?

KRAMER WAS INITIALLY MET with resistance from the psychiatric establishment. Many academic leaders had long been committed to Freudian psychotherapy; they had resisted for years the notion of using medications even for severe mental illnesses like schizophrenia. The notion of using medications even for mild anxiety and depressive symptoms—the millions of "worried well" people who represented the bread-and-butter of psychotherapy practice—was anathema to them. Others, who practiced psychopharmacology, were committed to the medical model: they wanted to treat disease in very sick people, not to make the entire population happy and enlightened.

Almost twenty years later, despite this initial resistance, we have to grant that Kramer's predictions have come true. We now live, as the psychiatrist David Healy describes it, in an "antidepressant era."

After all, who would not want to be better than well? In this highly competitive society, where work is so valued and material achievement prized, if a pill would give one more energy and a leg up on the guy next door, why not use it? As Kramer put it, "[In] today's high-tech capitalism . . . confidence, flexibility, quickness, and energy . . . are at a premium." In fact, there has been some speculation that part of the late 1990s stock bubble may have been driven by a high percentage of New York investors being hyped-up on Prozac and related antidepressants. Just like there is surgery for the sick and plastic surgery for the well, why not a psychopharmacology for the sick, and, as Kramer put it, a "cosmetic psychopharmacology" for the well?

Plastic surgery is reserved for a small minority of the population, though, partly because it is expensive and not paid for by medical insurance since it doesn't involve treating medical illness. Cosmetic psychopharmacology would have to be a different matter. Given that about 10 percent of the American population appears to meet criteria for severe clinical depression at some point in their lives, meaning about 25 million people, medical insurance coverage barely can handle those who are accepted as being ill. If we include the rest of the population, or most of it, as simply being unhappy in some way with their lives, it is obvious that cosmetic psychopharmacology treatment would have to involve the majority of the American population. Yet while the idea of cosmetic psychopharmacology is attractive to many people, the idea of paying out of pocket for it tends not to meet with favor among ordinary Americans.

Kramer's prediction came true with a twist. Instead of psychiatrists and citizens forthrightly saying that they sought to improve their normal state, and paying for it out of pocket, everyone colluded with a reframing of the concept of illness, which was broadened to include many with mild anxiety or depressive symptoms. If one didn't meet the full criteria for severe clinical depression, one might meet milder criteria for "dysthymia" or "generalized anxiety disorder" or "social anxiety disorder" or "late luteal-phase dysphoric disorder" (premenstrual syndrome) or perhaps something like "chronic fatigue syndrome" or "fibromyalgia" or, more recently, "adult attention deficit disorder."

These conditions happened to respond to Prozac or its cousins, according to various studies, and most antidepressants received official sanction from the Food and Drug Administration to treat these diagnostic labels.

Psychiatrist David Healy and others call this method "disease-mongering": instead of creating drugs to treat diseases, we create diseases for which we can use our drugs (see chapter 7). They blame the pharmaceutical industry for engaging in marketing, no different from any other kind of marketing. If I have a new cookie, and most people have not eaten it, I will advertise and create markets by encouraging people to try my new cookie, with the result, if I succeed, that eating my kind of cookie will now be a part of the American diet, where it was not previously. The pharmaceutical industry, Healy argues, has done the same with psychiatric illnesses, particularly depression and its varieties. Kramer too notes that many of us are influenced by a "pharmacocentric view of the world." In Western society today, drugs become both metaphors and mechanisms by which we understand and interpret our lives: Valium calmed the anxiety of the 1960s; Prozac spurred the acquisitiveness of the 1990s.

I think both Healy and Kramer are correct. Healy is right: the pharmaceutical industry clearly has manipulated the definitions of illness to its profit, and much of what is being treated with antidepressants is not psychiatric illness, certainly not in the severe forms that traditionally have been the center of clinical attention. Kramer is right: there is a great deal of psychological suffering out there, and psychiatric medications can help to alleviate some of that suffering, at least in some people.

Here's a solution to this apparent paradox: we have to distinguish between the depressive realism and the cognitive distortion models.

Mild levels of depressive symptoms actually produce insights that are useful for life

Where we're dealing with depressive realism, Healy is right; where we're dealing with cognitive distortion, Kramer is right. In other words, mild levels of depressive symptoms actually produce insights that are useful for life and can ultimately lead to greater happiness. On the one hand, trying to treat away these mild levels of depression, even if

---

More severe depressions impair insight and should be treated

---

we could, would ultimately be counterproductive in terms of happiness. More severe depressions, on the other hand, impair insight and should be treated, producing greater ability to live one's life fully.

As one of my patients once pointed out, treating away depression doesn't in itself produce happiness; it merely removes an obstacle, the illness of depression, that stands in our way on the path toward happiness.

THE QUESTION REMAINS WHAT to make of Kramer's claim that Prozac is useful in nondepressed persons with mild depressive and anxiety symptoms. If these persons have depressive realism, we would expect Prozac to be unhelpful. Yet Kramer clearly describes cases, six in all, where Prozac was quite useful.

Reading those cases is instructive. As Kramer points out, none of these persons has classic severe major depression. In classic depression, a person will have a normal personality, and then an episode of severe depression, which usually lasts about six to twelve months and then resolves spontaneously. For a number of years, one might be completely normal, happy as usual, average in one's mood and energy. Then another depression would occur, last six to twelve months, resolve, and so on. The persons in Kramer's cases did not have severe depressions that would meet standard psychiatric criteria for a full major depressive episode. Rather they had chronic mild sad mood, anxiety, marked shyness, and other personality features that interfered with success in relationships or at work and led to increased personal unhappiness. On Prozac, they became more outgoing, optimistic, and energetic, resulting in closer relationships with more people and greater achievements at work or in school.

In each case, Prozac was treating the individual's personality, or character, his or her ongoing baseline state of mood, energy, and attitudes. It's not surprising that there was some effect, since we know that personality, like everything else, has a biological component (though it's not completely biological). That biological component can be affected by Prozac or other medications in some cases. All personality lies on a normal curve; for instance, for the personality trait of introversion-extraversion, some people are highly introverted (very shy), some are highly extroverted (outgoing and bubbly), most are somewhere in between. Another major personality trait is anxiety, also called *neuroticism*: Some people are highly anxious (very nervous, worrywarts), some are hardly anxious (calm, Zen-like), most are somewhere in between. A few clinical studies show that serotonergic antidepressants, like Prozac, seem to shift personality traits up or down the normal curve that characterizes humankind. Thus, for instance, a less extroverted person becomes more extroverted or a more anxious/neurotic person becomes less anxious/neurotic. These kinds of personality changes are sometimes quite notable and independent of any effects on depressive symptoms per se. In this sense, the apparent conflict between Kramer and Healy may represent a confusion about what is being affected: an illness or a personality trait. If you are extremely introverted and anxious as your baseline personality, Prozac likely will help you. If you are extremely extroverted and calm, you hardly need it and it likely will not help you. For most of us, at or near the middle of the normal curve for personality traits, Prozac will be neither here nor there.

FOR MOST OF US normal, all too normal, people, there's no pill for happiness. Antidepressants aren't the solution. Though necessary for the minority of persons with severe clinical depression, or for those with marked extremes of personality traits, antidepressants like Prozac do not make most of us happier. In fact, mild depressive symptoms—what used to be called *melancholic temperament*—probably provide some insights into the realities of life that ultimately will guide us onto the path of happiness. An important step toward heading in the direction of real happiness is to give up the fantasy of pharmacological happiness. The reality is that just as our gadgets and toys are marketed to us, we have been marketed, by the pharmaceutical industry, into using many of our pills, especially the antidepressants. What is relevant here is not only that Prozac may not help with our daily unhappiness but rather that it might cause us to become even more unhappy by creating a manic response. American capitalism run amok directly seeks to cause manic superficiality in place of a real human reaction to our despair.

American capitalism run amok directly seeks to cause manic superficiality in place of a real human reaction to our despair

---

In other words, Prozac causes mania. We know this in patients with psychiatric illness. By mania, I mean the clinical syndrome of being highly hyperactive, not needing to sleep for weeks on end, speaking rapidly, and often doing impulsive things like spending a great deal of money or having sexual indiscretions. In persons with manic-depressive illness, we see these symptoms as part of that illness. In others who appear only to have severe depression, Prozac and other antidepressants can cause such manic periods.

One can see such clinical cases of Prozac-induced mania as an analogy to what is happening with the extensive use of antidepressants in the American population. Here I will also include the high use of amphetamine stimulants, like Ritalin, in children, since amphetamines also are antidepressants. The effect of Prozac and Ritalin given to millions of adults and children is to make them somewhat more hyperactive, in many cases, somewhat manic. Perhaps it is not surprising given our discussion of how America promotes a manic-like culture of superficial activity. Prozac and antidepressants feed into that kind of manic-like behavior, hence their popularity. But, if such manic superficiality is harmful, keeping us from being aware of the real despair of our lives, then the use of these antidepressants at a population-wide level is also harmful.

MARGARET STROLLED INTO MY office confidently: "Don't you dare give me any antidepressants!" she pronounced. "They all make me worse. That's why I came to you. Cure me."

Obviously, I wouldn't need to analyze the risks and benefits of antidepressants with her. She had taken them all, at least all the new ones, over about twenty years. Once, when she was taking Prozac, she stopped sleeping for two days, and then she began to feel a major surge in sexual energy. She got on her computer and e-mailed a colleague at work; he was married, so was she, but her sexual desire for him made the details of marriage seem puny.

"I must have sex with you," she wrote, going on in detail to describe what kinds of sexual activity she wished to engage in. Six hundred e-mails ensued over two weeks, followed by a business trip in which the liaison was consummated. She had been depressed, though she had never been suicidal or needed to be hospitalized. She had never experienced mania in the past. Her psychiatrists, four of them, over the course of those twenty years had diagnosed her with mild depression repeatedly, though curiously she never got more than a little better with her antidepressants, often only for a few months, and then inexplicably the down moods would return, she would feel somewhat fatigued, she couldn't concentrate too well, and she would be slower than others in her investment company. She needed to be on the top of her game: she needed antidepressants. (Many people get manic on antidepressants and then sink into depression afterward; they never get "well," meaning stably normal, and instead cycle more and more quickly into and out of depressive episodes.)

About a week after the hotel affair, she began to feel a little guilty. Her sexual appetite had changed from a gaping ocean of lust to a large river of desire. She saw her psychiatrist, asked him if what she had experienced was abnormal: her psychiatrist changed the antidepressant to another one.

Finally, her husband found out what had happened, and they both visited her psychotherapist. On her therapist's advice, she stopped her antidepressant and went back to her usual self, a little depressed but no longer manic.

After she saw me, we treated her with mood stabilizers that removed her mild depression and prevented mania as well. She was doing quite well for three years, yet she always said, in case I would forget, "Remember, don't ever give me an antidepressant."

And yet, we still do. About two-thirds of all prescriptions for psychiatric medications in the United States are for antidepressants. When we add neuroleptic (antipsychotic) drugs, also given for depression and mania, psychiatric medications are second only to cardiology drugs as the most profit-making class of drugs in the world (in 2006 global revenues were $13.1 billion, with cardiology drugs bringing in $18. 9 billion). Do so many people really need so many drugs? How do doctors rationalize all this prescribing?

To answer these questions, we should ask what it means to be a doctor. Usually, when we ask that question, we hear the ancient Greek medical thinker, Hippocrates, being referred to in a way that misunderstands what he taught.

CHAPTER 5

The Unknown Hippocrates

WE HAVE LOST THE LINK to the Hippocratic tradition in psychiatry today. We don't even know what it means. This would be like philosophers having forgotten about Plato, or Newton being misunderstood in modern physics, or Darwin being ignored in biology.

Hippocrates is not just a symbol; he was a profound philosopher of medicine; he taught us what medicine should be and the dangers of what it is. Wherever doctors have seriously thought about the meaning of their profession, the wisest of them are inevitably led back to the physician from Cos.

Most pay lip service to him and, if asked, will associate the man with the Hippocratic Oath and with the maxim "First do no harm." In fact, Hippocrates never said this; the phrase was invented in the mid-nineteenth century and falsely attributed to the Greek physician.

Despite its historical falsehood, if we ask what this maxim means, most physicians, never having taken a history of medicine course, will tend to reply that it means that one should not harm the patient, first and foremost. Or perhaps they will translate it into standard risk-benefit analysis, where the benefits of treatment should outweigh the harm.

This is all superficial.

It would be like physicists saying that Newton sat under a tree and taught us that things fall. There was much more to Newton than the law of gravity; there is much more to Hippocrates than the Hippocratic Oath.

PSYCHIATRISTS PRESCRIBE DRUGS FREQUENTLY. Do we have reason for concern? My view is that contemporary psychiatric practice far exceeds its scientific evidence base with overuse of psychotropic medications, contrary to the Hippocratic tradition (defined below). I don't argue that psychotropic medications should be avoided, nor simply prescribed less frequently, but rather they should be used within a consciously neo-Hippocratic philosophy (I say "neo" because I'm interpreting Hippocratic thinking for our era, not the fourth century BC). The best rationale for psychopharmacology—*when* to prescribe, when *not* to prescribe, *what* to prescribe—is to be found in a rediscovery of the Hippocratic approach to diagnosis and treatment.

In the United States, psychiatrists prescribe medications to 82 percent of their patients. From 1987 to 1997, use of antidepressant medications for depression doubled from 37 percent to 74 percent. Psychotherapy for such patients decreased slightly from 71 percent to 60 percent. Between 1987 and 1999, the use of antidepressants for anxiety disorders also increased from 18 percent to 44 percent. Benzodiazepine anti-anxiety medications (like Valium or Ativan or Klonopin) are also commonly prescribed; yet in 47 percent of cases, independent researchers could not identify diagnosis-based indications for such anxiolytics. In general, psychotherapy treatment has not decreased in frequency (3.2 per 100 persons in 1987 versus 3.6 per 100 in 1997), but psychotherapy alone is much less frequent (concomitant antidepressant use increased from 14 percent in persons receiving psychotherapy in 1987 to 49 percent in 1997).

This practice pattern is a major reversal compared with three decades ago, when most psychiatrists primarily practiced psychotherapy. A psychopharmacology revolution has occurred, abetted by advances in neurosciences and a shift in psychiatry toward greater emphasis on making diagnoses (as in the classic medical tradition) after the third edition of the American Psychiatric Association's *Diagnostic and Statistical Manual of Mental Disorders* (*DSM-III*) was published in 1980.

Where psychotherapies used to be seen as central, and often cu-
rative, decades ago, now psychopharmacology is seen as central to
psychiatric conditions like mood disorders, with psychotherapies as
adjunctive, although the combination sometimes is viewed as more
effective than either alone.

In theory, it is often stated that medications plus psychotherapies
provide optimal treatment, with the biopsychosocial model (see chapter 6) commonly invoked. In practice, psychotherapies are expensive or inaccessible to some patients; sometimes patients opt out of
psychotherapy based on their own preferences; often, insurance companies preferentially reimburse cheaper options (medications or psychotherapies provided by nonpsychiatrists). Given these scientific and
nonscientific factors, psychiatric medications are almost invariably
used, while psychotherapies are intermittently provided.

Also, there are the sobering results of the National Comorbidity
Survey: only about 50 percent of persons currently treated by clinicians (mostly with psychotropic medications) have a diagnosable mental disorder. In other words, psychiatrists practice treatment prompted
by symptoms rather than by diagnosis.

THE PRACTICE OF PSYCHIATRY today, then, involves aggressive treatment of symptoms with medications. Is this approach in the best scientific, ethical, and historical tradition of the medical profession?

There is a general misunderstanding of the term "Hippocratic,"
often associated with the ethical maxims of the Hippocratic Oath, such
as "First do no harm," later Latinized as *Primum non nocere*. A false
claim, as noted: The full original quote was in the maxim from Book
I of *Of the Epidemics*: "As to diseases, make a habit of two things—to
help, or at least to do no harm." The Hippocratic tradition in medicine is thus identified simply with a conservative approach to treatment. While partly true, this popular simplification fails to capture the
deeper genius of his thinking, for its ethical maxims were not abstract
opinions but rather grew out of the Hippocratic theory of disease.

The basic Hippocratic belief is that Nature is the source of healing and that the job of the physician is to aid Nature in the healing process. A non-Hippocratic view is that Nature is the source of disease and that the physician (and surgeon) needs to fight Nature to effect a cure. Even in ancient Greece, physicians had many potions and pills to cure ailments; Hippocrates resisted that interventionistic medicine, and his treatment recommendations often involved diet, exercise, and wine—all designed to strengthen natural forces in recovery. If Nature will cure, then the job of the physician is to hasten Nature's work carefully and to avoid adding to the burden of illness.

Based on this philosophy of disease, the followers of Hippocrates divided diseases into three types: curable, incurable, and self-limiting. *Curable* diseases require intervention, aimed at aiding the natural healing process. *Incurable* diseases generally were best left untreated, since treatments didn't improve illness and, due to side effects, would only add to suffering. *Self-limiting* diseases also didn't require treatment, since they improved spontaneously; by the time any benefits of treatment would occur, the illness would resolve by itself, again leaving only an unnecessary side effect burden. The concept of *Primum non nocere*, thus, meant knowing when to treat and when not to treat, based on what kind of disease one diagnosed.

IF APPLIED TO PSYCHOPHARMACOLOGY, a Hippocratic approach would avoid medications as much as possible, except where we can clearly help the natural process of healing and with great attention to side effects. A psychopharmacologist in the Hippocratic tradition

> *A Hippocratic approach would avoid medications as much*
> *as possible, except where we can clearly help the natural*
> *process of healing and with great attention to side effects*

prescribes less when the natural history of a mental illness involves spontaneous resolution at some point, as in mood episodes. The Hippocratic psychopharmacologist often would refrain from prescribing any medications at all, instead emphasizing psychosocial interventions—such as psychotherapies or lifestyle changes (moving, changing jobs, exercise)—to spur the natural healing process.

Non-Hippocratic approaches are best exemplified by the Galenic tradition, most associated with a belief that the body is ruled by four liquids, or humors, which were thought to affect both the emotions and physical health. In previous eras, fluids had to be kept "in balance" by bloodletting or inducing vomiting. (Now, keeping a balance of chemicals like serotonin or dopamine is the impetus behind diagnosis and treatment.) Clinical observation is demeaned. Nature is viewed as the Enemy, and the doctor as the source of the cure. Treatments are given freely, with the belief that illnesses will not abate otherwise.

THE HISTORY OF MEDICINE (including psychiatry) can be viewed as a constant conflict between Hippocratic and Galenic traditions. This dichotomy about nature and disease is somewhat artificial. Nature appears to be both cause of disease *and* source of healing. Indeed, with some diseases, a surgeon does cure disease, quite non-Hippocratically, by *cutting it out*. But, even in surgery, the Hippocratic tradition is central. For instance, current wound healing methods are the result of a long battle between Hippocratic ("God heals, and the surgeon dresses the wounds": keep the wound clean) and non-Hippocratic (repeated surgical debridement, which delays healing) views.

In the history of psychiatry, the contrast between these two philosophies has been constant. One can view "moral therapy," introduced by the late eighteenth-century French psychiatrist Philippe Pinel, as a return to Hippocratic methods (Pinel overtly viewed himself as Hippocratic). In contrast, his contemporary Benjamin Rush, the father of American psychiatry, directly and savagely attacked Hippocratic thinking for its therapeutic conservatism ("It is impossible to calculate the mischief which Hippocrates has done, by first marking Nature with his name, and afterwards letting her loose on sick people. Millions have perished by her hands.") Rush strongly advocated treating mental illness with extensive bleeding with leeches and purging by taking emetics. Some twentieth-century approaches to biological psychiatry, such as psychosurgery and colectomy cure of schizophrenia, are also non-Hippocratic theories. This history cannot be ignored. To move toward a new Hippocratic psychopharmacology for the twenty-first century, we should first learn from the great Hippocratic teachers of the nineteenth century.

LIKE HIPPOCRATES, THE CANADIAN physician William Osler, who was the famed chief of medicine at the Johns Hopkins Hospital at the turn of the twentieth century and later at Oxford, is often cited but little read. He is most known for his emphasis on patients as persons, as the father of medical humanism, the ideal well-bred physician. Yet in his prime, Osler was a cutting-edge scientifically oriented physician; he emphasized the importance of pathology and based clinical skills on pathological confirmation and laboratory testing. He is misinterpreted as a mere humanist and bedside clinician; he tested his clinical observations by what he saw when he conducted over a thousand autopsies. He strongly advocated the Hippocratic tradition, stressing clinical observation and diagnosis and opposing aggressive medication treatment. His therapeutic conservatism (some called it "nihilism") was not simply a personal attitude but, like Hippocrates, the upshot of scientific medicine.

In Osler's age, physicians had recently replaced bleeding and purging with pills and potions. Taking the Hippocratic view, Osler disapproved of those extensive treatments (both the bleeding and purging as well as the pills and potions) because they disregarded disease: "A man cannot become a competent surgeon without a full knowledge of human anatomy, and the physician without physiology and chemistry flounders along in an aimless fashion, never able to gain any accurate conception of disease, practicing a sort of popgun pharmacy, hitting now the malady and again the patient, he himself not knowing which."

Osler felt that scientific medicine is the treatment of diseases, not symptoms. Physicians needed to shift their focus from identifying and treating symptoms to understanding the diseases that cause those symptoms. Once those diseases were understood, Osler held, appropriate treatments would arise. Instead of anti-jaundice treatments for yellow skin, anti-pyretic treatments for fever, pro-energy treatments

for fatigue, and anti-chill treatments for coldness, the syndrome causing those symptoms needed to be studied and, if identified as a disease
(like hepatitis), treating the single disease would cure many symptoms.

In short, the solution was diagnosis before drugging:

> In the fight we have to wage incessantly against ignorance and quackery
> among the masses, and follies of all sorts among the classes, diagnosis,
> not drugging, is our chief weapon of offence. Lack of systematic personal
> training in the methods of the recognition of disease leads to the misap-
> plication of remedies, to long courses of treatment when treatment is use-
> less, and so directly to that lack of confidence in our methods which is apt
> to place us in the eyes of the public on a level with empirics and quacks.

This was the line of demarcation between scientific and nonscientific medicine. Nonscientific physicians asked only to know symptoms,
followed by treatments. Scientific physicians sought to know whether
symptoms led to disease, and only then might they treat the disease:

> The nineteenth century has witnessed a revolution in the treatment of
> disease, and the growth of a new school of medicine. The old schools—
> regular and homeopathic—put their trust in drugs, to give which was the
> alpha and omega of their practice. For every symptom there were a score
> or more medicines—vile, nauseous compounds in one case; bland, harm-
> less dilutions in the other. The characteristic of the new school is firm
> faith in a few good, well-tried drugs, little or none in the great mass of
> medicines still in general use.

Osler's reference to "a few good, well-tried drugs" is especially relevant to psychiatry. We have basically four major categories of drugs—
antidepressants, anti-anxiety medications, mood stabilizers, and antipsychotics—and, with a few exceptions, agents within each class are
of similar efficacy. Our most potent biological interventions have been
with us for many years: electroconvulsive therapy, or ECT (1938),
lithium (a mood stabilizer, 1949), monoamine oxidase inhibitors (antidepressants, 1957), benzodiazepines (anti-anxiety drugs, 1960), and
clozapine (an antipsychotic, 1963); no more efficacious drugs have
since been discovered in any of the four classes. (While an exaggera-

tion, the Canadian innovator in psychopharmacology Heinz Lehmann once said that with the oldest amphetamine, dextroamphetamine, and the first antipsychotic, chlorpromazine, he could treat all psychiatric conditions.)

Osler also foresaw future politics: if we reject disease-oriented medicine, we are left at the mercy of social forces tending toward overmedication: patients themselves ("Man has an inborn craving for medicine"); the pharmaceutical industry (about whom his warnings are all too familiar: "To modern pharmacy we owe much, and to pharmaceutical methods we shall owe much more in the future, but the profession has no more insidious foe than the large borderland pharmaceutical houses."); and doctors' own economic interest (giving pills keeps customers happy).

Thus we have the first rule for a Hippocratic psychopharmacology:

Osler's Rule: Treat diseases, not symptoms.

ANOTHER KEY FIGURE WHO fought non-Hippocratic medicine was Oliver Wendell Holmes, who, in an 1861 lecture to the Massachusetts Medical Society, described the role of medications in Hippocratic medicine:

> Presumptions are of vast importance in medicine, as in law. A man is presumed innocent until he is proven guilty. A medicine . . . should always be presumed to be hurtful. It always is *directly* hurtful; it may sometimes be *indirectly* beneficial. If this presumption were established . . . we should not so frequently hear the remark . . . that, on the whole, more harm than good is done by medication. (italics in original)

Holmes then proceeded to draw the conclusions that would follow:

> Throw out Opium, which the Creator himself seems to prescribe, for we often see the scarlet poppy growing in the cornfields, as if it were foreseen that wherever there is hunger to be fed there must also be pain to be soothed; throw out a few specifics [i.e., vitamins and minerals] which our art did not discover, and is hardly needed to apply; throw out wine, which is a food, and the vapors which produce the miracle of anesthesia, and I

firmly believe that if the whole material medica [equivalent to our current *Physician's Desk Reference*], *as now used,* could be sunk to the bottom of the sea, it would be all the better for mankind,—and all the worse for the fishes. (italics in original)

This eloquent plea for a return to Hippocratic principles in medicine made the front page of the *New York Times,* but it has failed to take root in modern medicine.

HOLMES CAN BE SEEN as simply presaging the notion of best practices for each individual patient found in evidence-based medicine: He requires proof that medications work before they are prescribed. In fact, Holmes's lecture was cited a century later to support the 1963 Food and Drug Administration (FDA) law requiring proof of efficacy to market medications in the United States.

Yet Holmes went further: he provided a philosophy of pharmacology. He argued that the baseline, default position of clinicians should be not to use medications (until proven effective), rather than having a default position to use medications (until proven harmful). This is a legalistic argument (appropriate for the father of a famed Supreme Court justice): In the law, a person is innocent until proven guilty; in medicine, according to Holmes, drugs should be guilty until proven innocent. There should be a presumption they are harmful. They need not be proven harmful; they *do* need to be proven safe and effective.

In Holmes's theory then, when physicians assess risks and benefits of a treatment, they need to start on the benefit side of the ledger. Since we presume all drugs to be harmful, none should be used until there is some proof of benefit (the more valid scientific proof, the better). The universe of options should be limited to proven treatments, not to all available (but often poorly proven) treatments. Instead, patients and physicians frequently begin on the safety side, asking: What are the safest available drugs? On this approach, placebo would be the safest treatment to use, or placebo-like drugs, quite benign in side effects but often rather ineffective (especially in off-label usage). An example is the extensive use of the anticonvulsant gabapentin for mood disorders in the late 1990s, despite its lack of proven efficacy at that time, followed by evidence of its inefficacy in acute mania.

So, a second rule for a Hippocratic psychopharmacology would then be:

Holmes's Rule: All medications are guilty until proven innocent.

TODAY MANY PSYCHIATRISTS PRACTICE nonscientific symptom-oriented treatment, giving sedatives for insomnia, stimulants for fatigue or distractibility, anxiolytics for tension, antidepressants for depressive symptoms, and mood stabilizers for mere moodiness—leading to an excessive and ineffective polypharmacy.

Critics will support symptom-oriented approaches because, they might say, we don't really understand mental illnesses as medical disease entities. We don't know their causes or their pathophysiology. But there are at least two well-established diseases in psychiatry: schizophrenia and manic-depressive illness. There is extensive research on their causes and pathophysiology, and even, in the case of bipolar disorder, a cure (lithium completely cures all symptoms in about one-third of such patients). We understand diseases much better now, after the neuroscience revolution, than we did previously. Even our lack of understanding supports this Hippocratic disease-based approach. The Hippocratic philosophy tells us what to do when we don't know about diseases, as well as when we do. When we don't know for sure if diseases are present, the tradition tells us *not* to treat. Critics will say that patients come to us for help; they are suffering; we have to do something; we must treat their symptoms. What Hippocrates teaches is that frequently not doing something is the best thing we can do. That's the meaning behind the maxim: As to diseases, try to help, or at least not to harm.

These ideas may prove less controversial if we understand the concept of a *diagnostic hierarchy*. Derived from the European tradition in psychiatry, the idea here is that certain diagnoses should not be made (those lower on the hierarchy) if other diagnoses are present (those higher on the hierarchy): *All diagnoses are not created equal.* So we shouldn't diagnose schizophrenia when someone hears a voice, unless depression and mania are first ruled out. Or, we shouldn't diagnose panic disorder, or "personality disorders," when someone is depressed. The same applies to other monosymptomatic diagnoses: ADHD, eating disorders, sexual addictions.

The concept of a diagnostic hierarchy is the basis of a Hippocratic approach to drug treatment. Since mood illnesses can produce not only depression and mania but almost *any* psychiatric symptom, treatment of mood conditions can improve all associated *non-mood* symptoms. Instead of many drugs for many symptoms, we would use one drug for the disease that causes many symptoms.

WE ARRIVE AT THE HIPPOCRATIC ethical conclusion of doing no harm *at the end*, not at the beginning. It is the result of treating disease, not symptoms. It isn't about the idea of avoiding treatments in general.

In the past, we avoided medications too much: psychoanalysis was seen as the solution. Now I believe we use medications too much: we practice a symptom-oriented psychopharmacology that belongs in the nineteenth century. We need to be clear about what we need to do: we should prescribe medications primarily for diseases, not symptoms, and not even for all diseases; we should avoid prescribing them by habit, only doing so when proof of benefit exists and far outweighs risks. With that basic philosophy, we can then turn to studies and research and data, leading to a scientific Hippocratic psychopharmacology. Otherwise, in my view, the science and the data are twisted by doctors and patients to their own whims, producing that eclectic mish-mash that is contemporary psychiatry. A rediscovery of the historically accurate Hippocratic method can permit modern psychiatry to get us closer to that ever-elusive, ancient goal of the school of Cos: *to cure sometimes, to heal often, and to console always.*

But before we can reach that goal, we have to distinguish true guides who can show us the way from pretenders who would send us on the wrong path.

II Pretenders

CHAPTER 6

Postmodernism Debunked

I BEGAN THIS BOOK by describing a dangerous way of thinking afoot in the land, a way of thinking so dangerous we don't even know we think this way. I'll now return to analyzing it in more detail, because those who pretend to lead us are commonly enacting ideas based on this ideology. This philosophy is assumed by the average American teenager and vigorously defended by the average American graduate student: it is postmodernism. In the context of this book, its claim is that there is no such thing as mood diseases. Or if there is such disease, it's not what we think it is.

By legislating away disease, postmodernist thinking relativizes everything, becoming a universal acid that dissolves all truths into nothingness, allowing for any or all ideas to be defensible. By adding the claim that all viewpoints are ultimately matters of power, postmodernism allows the Big Lie, repeated frequently and loudly enough, to become accepted as truth. In this way, despite its claim to being democratic and populist, postmodernist thinking is the royal road to totalitarianism, not just in political life but in the life of the mind.

Modern psychiatry, pretending to be smarter than the past, flashes a skepticism about knowledge, a sophistication that pretends to go beyond mere science. Postmodernism is not as complex a notion as might appear to some readers: one might initially be intimidated by all those French names (Foucault, Derrida, Lacan) and those long and numerous books. Perhaps the key notion behind postmodernism is most simply expressed by a recent critique of it by the senior Princeton philosopher Harry Frankfurt, titled *On Bullshit*. Frankfurt didn't use that term merely to heap abuse on postmodernism; he expresses,

---

Postmodernism allows the Big Lie, repeated frequently and loudly enough, to become accepted as truth

---

with notable philosophical seriousness, that postmodernism is all about bullshit, that is, the belief that all ideas are junk, merely means of persuasion, efforts to ideologize power; all this because there is no truth. We need have no special respect for words and ideas because they don't signify truth; words and ideas become bullshit.

Some will claim, mistakenly, that I'm being pejorative; I'm merely reporting the language that Frankfurt has used, a perspective widely shared by many sober philosophers, not to mention his many readers.

I FIRST EXAMINED how postmodernism came about culturally; now let's assess how it has evolved in psychiatry.

As Emerson said, philosophies can become part of our bones; we don't need to read thinkers to learn the ideas; when those ideas are part of the climate of cultural opinion, we imbibe them with our mothers' milk. Commentators have noted that one consequence of postmodernism is eclecticism. If there is no truth, and the world cannot be fundamentally altered in any "right" way, then any approach can make sense.

The specific form that this postmodernist eclecticism took in psychiatry came to be called the *biopsychosocial model*, also known by the abbreviation BPS. What this clumsy term really means has been the subject of much academic dissertation. Its use in medicine and psychiatry is generally attributed to a gastrointestinal doctor and psychoanalyst: George Engel. In the late 1970s, Engel advocated the BPS model as a way to get beyond sole reliance on biology in medicine (what he and many others call "biomedical reductionism"). There are psychological and social, not just biological, aspects to medical illness, he argued. This supremely rational suggestion was not new; but, in the 1970s, at the dawn of a new technological revolution in medical science, it struck a chord within general medicine and, more important, within the mental health professions. The barbarians at the gates were the pure scientists, the technicians with their microscope and gene arrays; the defenders of all that was good and holy were the psychotherapists (especially the favored Freudians among them). General medicine took note of their brother Engel's wishes: the BPS model became standard language in medical school curricula in the 1980s and onward. But the BPS concept really took root, and became holy writ, in the disciplines of psychiatry, psychology, and social work. After all, it proved that not only for mental illness, but for *all* illness, these professions were essential.

Engel wanted to psychologize medicine; the mental health workers who rallied around the BPS flag wanted to demedicalize psychiatry.

WHAT STARTED WITH SOME viable rationale was soon infected with the postmodern virus. The infection began when clinicians began to ask the question: Okay, given that all illness has biological, psychological, and social components, which should we emphasize in this case, for this patient, in these circumstances, with this condition? The BPS model provided no general answer to specific clinical questions. It was like saying the law of gravity exists but never being able to say how it specifically applied in the world to a physical object. Or, as some early critics suggested, it was like going to a restaurant to eat, and, instead of a menu, receiving a list of ingredients. One might admit that there are biological, psychological, and social ingredients to many illnesses, but in what combination? Are they always equally influential? Or should one prioritize one versus the others at times?

The BPS model had no ready answer, so clinicians improvised.

Their answer was *eclecticism*: anything goes; nothing is forbidden. I as a clinician may decide to emphasize psychotherapy; you as a patient may decide to focus on medications. Everyone is free to do whatever anyone wants to do, and there is no wrong answer. All answers are right.

If life were so simple, and all answers were correct, none of us would ever get a grade other than "A" in school, and all would graduate from Harvard and Oxford *summa cum laude*, and every man would indeed be a king. Life doesn't function that way, but psychiatry does.

Postmodernism devolves into one of two things: either all things are equally false, which produces nihilism; or all things are equally true, which produces eclecticism. In either case, people are left to fend

---

Either all things are equally false, which produces nihilism; or all things are equally true, which produces eclecticism. In either case, people are left to fend for themselves

---

for themselves. Some see this as freedom, or, perhaps, being doomed to be free: this nihilism is seen as acceptable because at least we are free. Instead, one might see it as anarchism, the freedom that only appears to be free because it is unlimited, which, in reality, leads to the enactment of the authoritarianism of the strong.

THE PRACTICAL IMPLICATIONS of postmodernist nihilism need to be highlighted. This kind of thinking arose before and after World War II: the Nazis first adopted its approach in formulating the Big Lie; since there is no objective truth, repetition would establish the truth as wished by the Fuhrer. There was no science, as George Orwell reminded us, only German Science and Jewish Science; hence the Fuhrer could determine what science was. In fact, Orwell's whole life work can be seen as a battle against the nihilism in thinking that abets and leads to totalitarianism. Heidegger was a Nazi for a time, and Nietzsche was the favorite philosopher of National Socialism. (This is not to say that those thinkers are evil; I am trying to show where their ideas played out historically.) Moral relativism allowed space for the banality of evil that led to Jewish genocide.

Nihilism lost the war but won the peace; the West became relativist, though mediated through American culture, as Allen Bloom persuasively explains. As he argues, post-Nazi nihilism became superficial and personal, rather than totalistic and political: "American nihilism is a mood, a mood of moodiness, a vague disquiet. It is nihilism without the abyss." Elsewhere Bloom writes: "We have here the peculiarly American way of digesting Continental despair. It is nihilism with a happy ending." But its political implications are not minor. We ought to keep in mind that this kind of postmodernist thinking is exactly opposed to the commitments of the Founding Fathers; if Americans seriously believe in the principles of the Revolution, if they really think Jefferson and Lincoln were right, then they must reject postmodernism.

Naturally, postmodernists become indignant when analogized to totalitarianism, claiming abuse of the fascist and communist epithets. Though a term be abused, its use isn't always abusive. There is real meaning to the concepts of fascism and totalitarianism.

And besides, this is not a matter of retrospective name-calling. Contemporaries to fascism made the critique of postmodernism I just described. Think about George Orwell, so much discussed, so little understood. Orwell was a democratic socialist, opposed both to communism and Nazism as well as to British conservatism. A central theme to Orwell's thinking is a rejection of postmodern nihilism. "The very concept of objective truth is fading from the world," he wrote, as he grieved what he saw as the death of truth. His example in that context was his experience in Spain during the 1930s civil war between fascists and leftists. Orwell was there, fighting on the side of the leftist Republic, composed of a tenuous alliance between Stalinists/communists and anarchists. The communists and anarchists hated each other, but they hated Franco more, hence their alliance. Orwell, more sympathetic to the anarchists than to the Stalinists, fell in with some anti-Stalinist brigades. Thin, starving, isolated, Orwell fought bravely, receiving wounds for his efforts. Orwell's anarchist friends valiantly fought Franco's soldiers; many died, many more were wounded, few survived untouched. Toward the end of the war, the Republic was dealt a death blow by the Soviet-Nazi pact of 1939. Overnight, the Stalinist communists went from fighting Franco to fighting the anarchists. The doomed anarchists were now pursued by two enemies. Orwell watched in horror as his former communist allies turned on his brave comrades; he barely escaped a massacre in which almost everyone he

knew was murdered, not by their fascist enemies but by their communist friends.

He stowed his way out of Spain, through France, passing time homeless in Paris, finally arrived back in England; he was a shell, emptied
of the ideals he had taken to Spain. He had seen the worst of humankind and the best. He got to work recording his experiences in his profound *Homage to Catalonia*. The image of those murdered comrades,
killed not by battle but by treason, never left him. The communists
in England, following the Soviet lead, denied any such massacre had
ever happened. In his memoir, Orwell wrote a detailed chapter, carefully documented, describing exactly what he saw, and using local news-
paper material to verify the communist-run massacres. His book editor
thought it was too much detail; it distracts from the story, he said, to put
so much material on an internal dispute of local leftist groups.

Orwell was unmoved. If he wrote nothing, the world might never
have known about the communist massacres: the Soviets and their
Western allies would have covered everything up; the truth would be
lost forever to history. No historian might ever find any documentation
to retrace what happened. How many such truths of human existence

---

*There is a type of human interaction that is based not on
knowledge, nor even lack of knowledge, but on failure to
know what isn't known*

---

have been lost to human history, Orwell wondered? Indeed the truth
could be demolished, destroyed, erased from human knowledge as if
it never existed. Orwell shuddered for us. We go through our lives not
knowing many things that no one knows about, which—some time,
some place—were real. John Kenneth Galbraith put it another way:
There is a type of human interaction that is based not on knowledge,
nor even lack of knowledge, but on failure to know what isn't known.

Postmodernism encourages attacks on truth, even revels in it; the
more truths are obscured and forgotten, the better postmodernists can
make their case that truths are all relative to power and culture and
that none of us have a better story to tell than anyone else. Orwell

knew better: He saw that this casual attitude toward truth allowed Stalinism to lie and pretend that its lies were truths; he saw that it allowed Nazism to sell its anti-Semitism. He saw a deep truth, perhaps the deepest: Once we allow all truths to be deconstructed away into nothingness, there will be no truths left to resist the Big Lie.

This postmodern disease has taken hold of all academia; the last redoubts are the sciences, and there the first to succumb has been clinical medicine, and within medicine, psychiatry.

ONE SYMPTOM OF POSTMODERNISM is the attack on the motivations of others. Commonly, motivations are presumed to be financial: everything is about money; hence postmodernists go on the warpath against the pharmaceutical industry and its collaborators in academic medicine. This belief comes across in recommendations such as that of Marcia Angell, former editor of the *New England Journal of Medicine* (and author of the soberly titled *The Truth about the Drug Companies: How They Deceive Us and What to Do about It*). Angell ends her book with recommendations that patients should ask their doctors whether they ever interacted at all with pharmaceutical companies, including receiving a pen or a note pad or giving lectures and receiving honoraria. If they had any such relationship ever, Angell recommends that patients should fire their doctors and get a new one! This would be like saying Americans should never vote for any politician who ever received a single dollar from any interest group. There would be no politicians for whom to vote.

Nihilism is also reflected in the Marxian adage so blithely pronounced by our anti-pharmaceutical sages (like Dr. John Abramson in his overheated tome *Overdosed America*): "Follow the money." In other words, if a researcher is funded by a pharmaceutical company, the study will be biased in favor of that company; any results produced by that research can be discounted as false. One also hears clinicians frequently say: "I don't know who to believe any more. One study says X, the other says the opposite; and they're always funded by opposing companies. I'll disbelieve them all." (And, they should admit, go on practicing based on their own, frequently false, opinions.)

The problem is that as a physician, you're not supposed to believe anyone. You are supposed to assess the evidence yourself and make an informed judgment, based on your two decades' worth of formal education. Now you may say that physicians cannot be expected to understand the statistical details of medical research. This would be like saying that physicians can't be expected to understand the physiological details of kidney function. You can't be a physician unless you have basic knowledge relevant to medical practice or unless you are able to augment your basic knowledge with further knowledge as experience and practice demand. Medical statistics is part of medicine now, and no physician is competent who doesn't have basic understanding of it.

Back to postmodernism: If you say that money solely drives data, and you completely ignore the content of research, then you are reducing research to money. There is no truth to the research that is being done; it's all about making a buck. Similarly if you say that a physician's competence is nullified by pharmaceutical associations, you are saying that he has no inherent abilities that he can ethically put into practice; it's all about making a buck.

The reason so many patients and clinicians can think this way is because they have become nihilists; they no longer believe in objective truths; everything is a relative combat between interest groups seeking power and wealth. This is the core idea of postmodernist thinking: it's all about money and power only if you place no value on anything else, namely objective truth. A lithium level of 4.0 is toxic and kills. This is a truth that is not relative or a matter of opinion; medical practice, at least, shows that postmodernism is false. A truth is not a lie when a patient dies. If we accept that simple fact—that there are truths that cannot be reduced to power and money—then we must reject all simplistic critiques of the pharmaceutical industry and of academic medicine.

Still the pharmaceutical industry and academic medicine both deserve a thorough critique. One extreme and the other are equally false: can we hit the truth in between?

CHAPTER 7

Pharmageddon?

THE UPSURGE OF POSTMODERNISM in our culture is manifested in psychiatry by concerted attacks on drugs and biological approaches. Frequently, some of those who support existential and humanistic approaches to psychology and psychiatry feel a need to go on a rampage against anyone who takes the "opposite" approach of biological or drug-based psychiatry. Myriads of books and articles attack the pharmaceutical industry, those who work with the pharmaceutical industry, those who live next door to the pharmaceutical industry, and their second cousins too.

There is no need for all of this bile.

But since it is there, one must be explicit in trying to understand what it is all about and trying to make some sense of it all. To give my conclusion first, I do not see why we cannot be both existential/humanistic and biological at the same time. In fact, I advocate a *biological existentialism*, which means that science and humanism, each properly understood, are not in conflict. Yet we misunderstand both.

A PROMINENT CRITIC in this vein is the psychiatrist David Healy. Coming from within the profession, a psychiatrist who has himself conducted psychopharmacology research, his critiques have carried some weight. He also has done the hard work of oral history in psychopharmacology, doing for this field what great historians like my friend Paul Roazen did for psychoanalysis (see chapter 13). There is no history without interpretation, and Healy's histories, though often well-documented and dispassionately presented, ultimately end in pas-

---

I advocate a **biological existentialism**, *which means that science and humanism are not in conflict*

---

sionate interpretations and prescriptions that are, in the end, one of multiple interpretations. Previously, he had criticized antidepressants, later antipsychotics, and, by extension, the psychiatric profession's current views regarding depression and schizophrenia. Here I will critique his ideas on bipolar disorder.

Healy writes: "Manic-depressive illness provides a compelling symbol of the current problems in medicine. Its dominant therapies are classified under an advertising rubric—mood stabilization. The core illness has been rebranded in a way that is all but meaningless. The basis on which its leading drugs were patented appears to make a mockery of the patent system, in terms of the goals of both novelty and public utility that the system is supposed to serve." This is his main idea. Is it right?

Healy shares the postmodernist assumption that medicine (and science) is not the progressive, simple affair it has seemed but rather a complex cultural construction. To him, not only the profession, but the illnesses themselves, are "social constructions." There is either no "real" entity out there that underlies these constructions, or, if there is, such a real entity is not the same thing as the varied cultural constructions that have existed over the years. The relevance of social, political, and economic factors for all human activity was insisted on long before Healy or Foucault; of course, Marx deserves due credit here. (I am not implying that this is good or bad, though perhaps some credit is due to Marx the thinker despite our cultural antagonism to Marxism.) This restatement of an old and true proposition still seems to sting, especially in what Healy terms today's American "corporate psychiatry." The proposition is old because Marx made it long before postmodernism existed; and true because not every illness is a biological disease; Marx long ago showed that social and economic factors influence human beliefs, often unconsciously. Some postmodernist ideas can be true, like these, but they tend to predate postmodernism. I am not claiming that all postmodernist ideas are false, but allowing for some to be true does not mean that postmodernism is inherently true either. An analogy would be to astrology: some ideas about which planets exist where are true; but the overall philosophy is false.

Healy is particularly bothered by the extension of bipolar diagnosis to children and inappropriate (sometimes fatal) use of psychotropic medications. That is not all there is to his critique, but it seems to be where the passion lies. Unhappiness with the extension of a diagnosis isn't a criticism of the diagnosis itself.

While some of these concerns may be valid, critics of psychiatric drugs often ignore evidence of their benefits. For instance, Healy hardly

---

Critics of psychiatric drugs often ignore evidence of their benefits

---

comments on the extensive literature demonstrating lithium's benefits in prevention of suicide and reduction of mortality—a clear medical outcome that challenges his implication that most psychiatric diagnoses and treatments are conducted on subjective grounds.

If Healy concludes that mood stabilizers like lithium are just "marketing fictions," then fiction will have to account for cases such as this one: Recently I consulted on a legal case of a 70-year-old man with bipolar disorder who had been completely stable and free of any mood symptoms at all for more than three decades. He was completely cured, while previously he had experienced severe suicidal major depressive episodes that didn't even respond to electroconvulsive therapy, a procedure once in common use and now the treatment of last resort for depression that doesn't respond to medications. He and his psychiatrist decided that, after so much wellness, perhaps he did not need lithium. Five months later, he had a new severe depressive episode and committed suicide. Apparently, the use of a marketing fiction for a meaninglessly defined entity cured, and its removal killed, this person.

TURNING FROM SCIENCE to history, Healy is particularly critical of those who claim that bipolar concepts are ancient. He wishes to counteract the assertion that ancient Roman or Greek physicians described anything similar to present-day bipolar disorder. To do this, he focuses on their description of physical signs, as opposed to subjective psychological emotions, and emphasizes the age-old commitment to the theory of four humors. Yet even with those aspects, it is difficult not to see the mania and melancholia of Hippocrates and first-century AD physician Aretaeus as having *some* similarities to today's mania and depression (even if differential diagnoses have changed and social construction is granted). These links are not lightly made but are based on translations from the original Latin made by European bipolar experts themselves. Healy's work is based on his own translations from the Greek; he feels that these other authors are selectively misrepresenting sections of the original Hippocratic works.

Declaring who is correct here will depend on further scholarship. But even if we grant that something like today's bipolar disorder was never described until mid-nineteenth-century France—which is Healy's view—then we also need to be explicit that pharmaceutical companies were nowhere to be seen in nineteenth-century France. Perhaps he is not arguing that bipolar disorder does not exist, that it is a fiction; rather, he seems to be saying that our current social construction of it is too broad. Nevertheless, I have already had one mental health professional gleefully cite Healy's book in the claim that the disorder is altogether a fiction, created by the pharmaceutical industry. Such readers at least need to provide the name of the pharmaceutical company so involved in 1854 Paris when physicians Jules Falret and Jules Baillarger first described the disorder.

Even the ghost of Emil Kraepelin is dishonored. Healy argues that Kraepelin's contribution was mainly in his definition of dementia praecox (DP; see chapter 2), and that his concept of manic-depressive insanity (MDI) is just a foil for nonspecific leftovers of DP. In fact, Kraepelin spent a good deal of effort and space in his descriptions of MDI, and he diagnosed and treated many such patients, many more than patients with DP. This is a matter of fact, not opinion; here are the results of an examination of medical records in Kraepelin's Munich clinic: In 1908, of 721 patients admitted, the most common diagnosis was alcoholism (161), followed by MDI (134); dementia praecox was seventh (53). Thus Kraepelin diagnosed MDI most frequently among primary psychiatric conditions and two and a half times more frequently than he did dementia praecox. Further, contemporary rediagnosis of those charts demonstrated that 23 percent of Kraepelin's MDI diagnoses would not meet current bipolar definitions: Kraepelin's view of MDI was that it was a broadly diagnosed and common condition. Healy's historical scholarship is simply mistaken. Kraepelin's main interest, clinically and theoretically, was in MDI; DP was not privileged in his thinking at all.

The concept of a recurrent mental illness, with highs and lows of mood, activity, and thinking (or mania and depression in current terms) has been around since before the mid-nineteenth-century French originators of bipolar disorder. Philippe Pinel described this condition (*periodic insanity*) as a core mental illness, in the very first pages of his 1806 *Treatise on Insanity*: "Intermittent or periodical insanity is the most common form of the disease. The symptoms which mark its accessions correspond with those of continued mania. Its paroxysms are of a determined duration, and it is not difficult to observe their progress, their highest development, and their termination." Pinel goes on to expound his moral treatment specifically for this disease, which approximates Kraepelin's MDI. Healy has recently translated Pinel's treatise from the French and draws the opposite interpretation about bipolar disorder. But as Healy himself admits, periodicity of abnormal behavior of the insane was clearly there in Pinel. The only question is whether we wish to diagnose this condition broadly, as Kraepelin did, as a recurrent disorder of mood, thought, and behavior—indeed as current advocates of a broad bipolar spectrum do—or whether we want to divide it up into many conditions (unipolar, bipolar, anxiety disorders), as *DSM-III* did.

HEALY MAKES A GREAT DEAL of how he believes Kraepelin would have been bothered by current "neo-Kraepelinian" efforts to revise and expand the bipolar concept in his name, even though Kraepelin's own MDI concept emphasized that the most common presentations were mixed mood states and mild temperament symptoms, not classic mania and melancholia. Current views of a broad bipolar "spectrum" are not new; Kraepelin's views were old and broad; in 1980, the American Psychiatric Association's *DSM-III* moved away from Kraepelin and toward the narrow nineteenth-century French concept of bipolar disorder. There it took the approach of the German psychiatrist, Karl Leonhard, who opposed Kraepelin's views and argued that MDI should be divided into two groups: unipolar and bipolar illnesses. Thus, *DSM-III* is not Kraepelinian, but Leonhardian, about mood disorders.

Healy has the wrong target: he seeks to deconstruct mania, thereby to dethrone bipolar disorder. Nowhere does Healy arrive clearly at the core of Kraepelin's concept of MDI. Manic-depressive illness (the non-French, non–*DSM-III* variety; the Kraepelin variety) is not defined by mania but rather recurrence of mood episodes (depressive *or* manic).

Current bipolar spectrum concepts are essentially trying to go behind *DSM-III* in history, back to the Kraepelinian, as opposed to the Leonhardian, paradigm, the exact opposite of "co-opting the Kraepelinian brand" to "move psychiatry into a world that Kraepelin would not recognize," as Healy claims. As an historical matter, Kraepelin's charts and his diagnostic practice are the opposite of the *DSM-III* bipolar conception, and current spectrum concepts are similar to Kraepelin's documented clinical world.

ANOTHER HEALYAN REPROACH to contemporary psychiatry is that the current view of mania and bipolar disorder is being broadened beyond the "core" condition unjustly. This critique is tautological:

he defines the core condition narrowly, following the current main-stream *DSM-III*–based view (following Leonhard and in line with pre-Kraepelinian notions in mid-nineteenth-century France); thus of course he would find few cases of a narrowly defined disease (as he shows based on late nineteenth-century records in Wales assessed using these criteria). But this critique begs the question, for it doesn't invalidate a broad view of mania: it merely shows that assessed narrowly, the condition is infrequent, and assessed broadly, it is frequent. Which approach is valid isn't addressed. Healy and others (like his contemporary, Peruvian psychiatrist German Berrios, whom he cites) may oppose broad use of the terms "mania" or "bipolar disorder," but this is itself an opinion, one among others. It is for clinical research to define the merits and flaws of the narrow versus broad interpretations, and that research, thus far, has shown a number of merits to the broad view (such as some supportive genetic, course, and treatment studies), as well as some weaknesses (including lack of consensus on its definition). Healy has assumed the weaknesses without giving much attention to the merits.

The assumption of inappropriate broadening of bipolar diagnosis occurs in a selective empirical vacuum: Healy doesn't cite an extensive underdiagnosis literature in recent years, which persists despite all the broadening of diagnosis in past decades. In the absence of empirical proof of mistaken diagnosis, one cannot presume that increased diagnosis represents increased *mis*diagnosis. AIDS also is diagnosed much more these days than it was in the 1980s.

The most important aspect of Healy's work is its underlying philosophy. It is a postmodernist interpretation of psychiatry, through and through. This is not to imply that Healy has read and studied Foucault or postmodern theory; it is to say that our culture is infected with these ideas. Karl Jaspers taught that we always ascribe to a philosophy, consciously or unconsciously. The world of Foucault has seeped into our culture, so that many of us in the Western world have imbibed these dogmas in our bones.

When one deconstructs bipolar disorder almost into nothingness, the question can be asked whether there is any practical difference between making the condition rare and narrowly defined versus simply viewing it as a fiction, a cultural artifact. If we replace biological with cultural reductionism, have we done anything meaningful?

THIS OEUVRE OF ANTI-PHARMACEUTICAL industry history, recently called "pharmageddon," is one of a growing genre, some of which is true, and some of which is less so.

A recent contribution that has some sense in it comes from Charles Barber. With extensive experience as a counselor to homeless mentally ill persons, Barber knows there is such a thing as serious psychiatric disease; his critique is not against medications in general or biological psychiatry per se. Rather, he thinks things are being overdone, and medications are used in those without mental illnesses in a manner that is not effective and perhaps harmful. Recall the recent epidemiological study that found that about half of all persons diagnosable with mental illness were not currently in treatment, but also that about half of persons currently in treatment were not diagnosable with current mental illnesses. Barber's critique isn't the one-sided claim that psychiatry is overmedicating everyone, but rather that the wrong people are getting medicated.

This question is more interesting to me than the increasingly well-worn generic critiques of the pharmaceutical industry and biological psychiatry. Since antidepressants are the most commonly prescribed psychiatric medications, these debates are often framed around those who are pro-antidepressant (such as Peter Kramer) versus those who are anti-antidepressant (such as Carl Elliott and Allan Horwitz and Jerome Wakefield, among others). The anti-antidepressant books seem to outnumber the pro-antidepressant books, with Peter Kramer a central target: Barber writes, for instance, that we should be listening to patients, not Prozac. Yet Kramer's point was that after years of listening to patients in psychotherapy, he achieved more success for their character traits after giving them Prozac. "Nobody writes about Prozac like that anymore!," notes Barber as he argues that a massive change happened in the 1990s, whereby antidepressant use surged and the biological approach to psychiatry took over our culture. Perhaps.

But the matter is not simple; I saw this transition in my own career: Psychiatry seemed quite biological to me in 1991 when I first entered the field, and it is still so. We used a lot of medications then. We still do; they just have different names. The implication that Kramer is something like a psychopharmacological Luddite conflicts with my experience that there is still a lot of interest in Prozac and antidepressants among most psychiatric practitioners in the "real" world (i.e., outside of academia), many of whom saw the limits of the psychotherapy era in prior decades.

The nuanced critique is this: if we grant the utility of antidepressants for severe depression, we can still critique their widespread usage for "subsyndromal depression" in Barber's phrase, or "community nervousness" as Healy puts it. This basic misery of human life is

---

This basic misery of human life is an existential, not a medical, fact

---

an existential, not a medical, fact, and Americans are culturally prone to trying to medicate it away. There is truth to this interpretation. What might be added is that such concepts were legislated away with *DSM-III* in 1980, when "neurotic depression" was removed from our diagnostic lexicon (see the next chapter): Only "major depressive disorder" was left (with a compromise to create "dysthymia" and "generalized anxiety disorder" to partially capture the prior neurotic depression group). After 1980, one had to reinterpret any depression as "major" depression; the move to widespread antidepressant usage only awaited drugs that were safe in overdose, the first of which was Prozac. A major reason why the class preceding Prozac, the tricyclic antidepressants, TCAs, were not widely prescribed by doctors was that if patients overdosed on the TCAs, they often died of cardiac arrhythmia. One can take hundreds of Prozac pills with no medical harm. This made the average doctor, sensitive to malpractice risks, much more comfortable with prescribing the new serotonin reuptake inhibitors. Now with two decades of research, we can conclude that antidepressants have little if any efficacy in neurotic (or mild) depression, justifying a return to using that diagnostic label so as to differentiate those with depression severe enough to need antidepressants from those who don't benefit for their mild symptoms.

Confusion and the constant debate about psychiatric drugs continue, partly because of the ongoing effects of our cultural postmodernism and its concomitant unwillingness to take science seriously. We need to explicitly discuss and critique this postmodernism if we ever hope to get our history right and understand the benefits and not just the harms of medications. Besides drugs, another way to understand these debates is to focus on diagnosis, especially that goliath of psychiatric diagnosis, "major depressive disorder." It is there that we need to go next if we are to unmask the pretenders from the guides in the world of depression.

CHAPTER 8

Creating Major
Depressive Disorder

THE HISTORIAN EDWARD SHORTER is a guide, not a pretender, though sometimes fallibly so. His research is central if we are to understand that psychiatric behemoth, major depressive disorder.

Shorter went to the American Psychiatric Association archives and dug up entertaining and informative minutes of many of the proceedings of the task force charged with preparing a new third edition of the *DSM* in the 1970s; he interviewed Robert Spitzer, the chairman of that task force, and others involved in the process. Shorter also read up on the Food and Drug Administration committee notes about the new generation antidepressants in the 1980s and 1990s, as well as earlier FDA records.

With this scholarship, he nicely reconstructs the debate about whether to include the concept of "neurotic depression" in *DSM-III*; how the term "minor" depression was rejected as implying that the illness was, well, minor; how the term "major" depression was created in the end to capture some of these milder kinds of depressions as well as the more severe melancholic version that had originally been intended; how psychoanalysts rebelled at the last second to preserve their livelihoods based on insurance reimbursement for neurotic depression; and how a "neurotic peace treaty" was devised whereby the terms "dysthymia" and "generalized anxiety disorder" were invented to allow psychotherapists something to bill.

He also describes the subsequent exploitation of *DSM-III* by the pharmaceutical industry in marketing serotonin reuptake inhibitors (SRIs). The stage was set in the 1960s and 1970s by the FDA's new rules, which legitimized the evidence-based medicine (EBM) movement, with its emphasis on clinical, rather than biological, research. Using meeting archives, he describes how the FDA moved from being hostile to the pharmaceutical industry in the 1960s and 1970s to being compliant with it in the 1980s and 1990s. He concludes that the FDA's later obsession with the so-called average effects seen in randomized clinical trials (RCTs) produced a "regulatory nihilism" whereby all negative studies were discounted and small positive effects were exaggerated in importance. For instance, having required two positive studies versus placebo for approval, the FDA ignored all negative studies. With Prozac, for instance, six of eight studies were negative. With Zoloft, all inpatient studies were negative; the drug was solely approved based on a few positive outpatient studies, the FDA knowing full well that it would also be used in hospitals, despite proof it didn't work in those patients. Worse, such negative studies usually went unpublished, and thus clinicians didn't know that they were using disproven agents in certain settings. A recent analysis of the FDA database found that published RCTs with new antidepressants produced about a 95 percent positive to 5 percent negative ratio; but once unpublished RCTs available at the FDA are included, the actual ratio is 51 percent positive to 49 percent negative.

As a non-clinician, Shorter holds views that are based to some extent on his clinical consultants, including David Healy, who represent a specific ideology in psychiatry, as discussed in the previous chapter. These clinicians support electroconvulsive therapy (ECT) as the most effective treatment in psychiatry. They are critical of most psychiatric diagnoses as now used, especially depression and bipolar disorder, as well as of the EBM movement. They think that such socially constructed concepts should be replaced by more biologically solid notions, like the old syndrome of "melancholia," a severe condition of depression with physical stereotyped symptoms (especially slowness of movement), biological correlates (marked overactivity of the adrenal gland reflected in a positive dexamethasone suppression test, DST), and most significant, excellent responsiveness to ECT but poor response to the Prozac-like SRIs.

There are scientific and historical problems with these beliefs.

Scientifically, the test of the adrenal grand, DST, has not been proven specific to melancholia. It may instead be mainly a marker of severity. More important, to privilege biological over clinical research is a Galenic move that itself has been disproven by the history of medicine. Galenic theory, based on the best biology of its time, held back medical progress (one must insist on the word) for two millennia. It led to bleeding and purging and much more harm than good, until it was disproven by . . . clinical research, statistics, the mid-nineteenth-century French physician Pierre Louis's "numerical method," all of which later led to randomized clinical trials and clinical epidemiology—the foundation of what is now called EBM. There is a case to be made against EBM, but there is also a strong case for it, both scientifically and historically.

IT MAY TURN OUT that melancholia as a syndrome is not, contrary to Shorter's beliefs, diagnostically important. To restate an important historical point: It was the view of Kraepelin (which Pinel presaged by several decades) that *recurrence* was the hallmark of a condition like manic-depressive illness, not the specific poles of melancholia and mania. This concept has some biological support (e.g., circadian

---

Recurrence was the hallmark of a condition like manic-depressive illness, not the specific poles of melancholia and mania

---

rhythm research), and it is completely ignored in much of the writing of this group of clinicians and historians (e.g., Healy's book on the history of bipolar disorder). If recurrence is the key aspect of this condition, then the diagnosis of manic-depressive illness would be more clinically and scientifically valid than the pathological state of melancholia (or mania).

Regarding electroconvulsive therapy, the matter is much more complex than simply viewing it as the most superior treatment for almost any psychiatric condition, including melancholia and mania. ECT is only a superior treatment in the short term; it has never been shown to be better than anything else long term, based on randomized data. Recently, the largest randomized clinical trial of maintenance ECT found that it was *not* more effective than antidepressant drugs plus lithium, despite the fact that the patients in that study were selected because they failed to respond to multiple antidepressant treatments. My understanding is that in earlier days (1960s and 1970s), ECT specialists used that method of treating mental illness only acutely, and they used lithium for long-term prophylaxis (not just for depressive but also for manic episodes; in the Kraepelinian view that they were preventing recurrence, with polarity being unimportant). That is how ECT was useful: to rapidly generate a normal mood, at which time one could then put the patient back on lithium prophylactically.

In contrast, ECT in recent years has been more widely used for ideological and economic reasons: Ideologically, doctors have become lax about diagnosis, or believe postmodernistically that clinical diagnoses do not matter; this belief in the unimportance of clinical diagnosis is then used to justify the nonspecific use and benefit of ECT for everything (depression, mania, psychosis). Economically, managed care insurance companies don't question weeks of hospitalization for ECT, whereas they breathe down doctors' necks when patients are only receiving medications. Frequently, patients get discharged without careful diagnosis, without any thought-through long-term drug prophylaxis, and end up either rehospitalized once ECT wears off or are committed to maintenance ECT largely by default. I have no problem with the acute use of ECT, if combined with careful clinical diagnosis, and good long-term drug prophylaxis, especially with mood stabilizers. This is how it is practiced by Italian mood disorder specialists, like Athanasios Koukopoulos in Rome and his group, who see themselves as inheritors of the mantle of one of the founders of this type of therapy in the 1930s, Lucio Bini. But by demeaning drugs to mere artifacts of EBM plus pharmaceutical marketing, ECT is left as only a short-term fix that guarantees long-term relapse.

There is much that is wrong with *DSM-III* and the way that it classifies depression and much that is mistaken in our use of new antidepressants. The concept of neurosis needs to be reconsidered and rehabilitated; the notion of melancholic depression is important; our antidepressant treatments are less effective in many ways than claimed. But ECT is not the cure-all, biological research is not more sound than clinical research, and replacing disease nosology with psychopathology, like melancholia, will not entail our mellifluous manumission from all this mistaken misery.

We are still left with the dilemma: Why are our psychiatric diagnoses, like MDD, so often bloated, and how can we get to a scientifically honest diagnostic system? We still have more history to learn first before we can answer these questions.

CHAPTER 9

The *DSM* Wars

TO UNDERSTAND WHY WE overdiagnose and mistreat depression, we have to understand major depressive disorder, or MDD; and to understand MDD we have to better understand the entire current system of psychiatric diagnosis, the *Diagnostic and Statistical Manual of Mental Disorders* (*DSM*).

The *DSM* was first published in the 1950s as an outgrowth of manuals used by the U.S. armed forces and the World Health Organization's *International Statistical Classification of Diseases* (*ICD*) and was then revised in the late 1960s. Our current *DSM* system is largely based on the third revision, *DSM-III*, which was published in 1980 and was, in many ways, a scientific advance. With it, American psychiatry moved from pure psychoanalytic ideology to at least some science.

Many see the fourth revision, *DSM-IV*, published in 1994, as a mere incremental advance on *DSM-III*. I used to think so as well. But I've come to the conclusion that *DSM-IV* was quite different; it marked a major change in how psychiatric leaders conceived diagnosis. In the process, it became a major problem for psychiatry as a profession in the past two decades.

This change became clear to me in the recent transition to *DSM-5*, which has been highly criticized by some of the leaders of *DSM-IV*. In the course of these debates, I was surprised to hear postmodernist-sounding arguments from some of those past leaders of *DSM-IV*: Science matters least, they say; our science is weak and debatable; pragmatic considerations should drive psychiatric diagnosis. I was further surprised to find that this line of reasoning was congenial to many colleagues in the profession, not to mention many in the public. One prominent science journalist from U.S. National Public Radio (NPR) told me that she had come to the conclusion that scientists are no different from anyone else; they just use "science" as a weapon to advance their opinions.

THE EXAMPLE OF BIPOLAR disorder is useful, I think, because it is one case where scientific evidence is reasonably present.

The scientific method for identifying different diseases in all of medicine, when one does not have a gold standard definition (such as an organ tissue sample), is information from different lines of evidence. The standard approach in diagnostic research in psychiatry, laid down in a classic article by Eli Robins and Samuel Guze, identifies those lines of evidence in five categories: symptoms (phenomenology), family history (which reflects genetic risk), course of illness (age of onset of symptoms, number of episodes, outcome), biological markers (which have not panned out as diagnostically specific in the intervening years of research), and treatment effects (reactions to certain medications that sometimes differ between diseases).

This research has been conducted with manic symptoms. In a very large and prospective thirty-year study conducted in the early 1990s, it was shown that two days of such symptoms were enough to differentiate two groups of persons (bipolar disorder type II vs. major depressive disorder). Increasing observation to four days didn't have any greater sensitivity or specificity for diagnosis. But these data have been ignored until now in favor of the pragmatic concern that, if the diagnosis of bipolar disorder was expanded, then it would become overdiagnosed and antipsychotics would be overused.

Let's imagine a thought experiment: Suppose we are like gods. (Many physicians are said to suffer from this delusion; here it is meant as a thought experiment.) As gods, since we know everything, we know that a certain disease exists. Let's call it disease X; in this disease, initial symptoms Y last two to three days, followed by other severe symptoms Z, which last weeks to months, eventually leading to death, if repeated, in 5 percent of persons.

Let's further suppose that doctors, being fallible human beings rather than god-like, mistakenly diagnose that disease only when its initial symptoms last four days or longer. Let's also suppose that no known effective treatments exist yet in the world.

Would the presence or absence of treatments make any difference as to the reality of the disease?

The reality of a disease is what it is, irrespective of what treatments may or may not be available, and irrespective of what human beings think.

There are, and always have been, many diseases in medicine for which no treatments have been available, but it has always still been useful for doctors to understand them as well as they can; treatments are often later developed.

Limitation in treatment doesn't justify ignorance of disease.

SOME NOSOLOGISTS TROT OUT the old threat of overdiagnosis despite another two decades of research repeatedly showing that bipolar disorder is actually underdiagnosed in about 30 to 40 percent of persons who have it. In those direct comparisons with major depressive disorder, bipolar disorder is underdiagnosed, while MDD is overdiagnosed. Even in reported claims of bipolar overdiagnosis, the data from those same studies show that bipolar disorder is twice more frequently underdiagnosed than overdiagnosed. The overdiagnosis fear (which underlies much of the concerns expressed by critics as reviewed in chapter 7) doesn't stand up to scientific scrutiny.

We are left with drug side effects. I agree that antipsychotics are overused but also think that antidepressants are overused. Why is it better to use antidepressants excessively in persons who don't have an illness that antidepressants treat (i.e., bipolar disorder; especially when we now know that antidepressants can also worsen that very illness)?

In a recent large analysis of practice patterns in the United States, mood stabilizers—lithium, valproate, carbamazepine—are in fact the least frequently used class of psychotropic medications and the only class whose use has not increased in the past decade.

The drug fear is overstated.

Even if we had no drugs, though, the point is irrelevant to the reality of trying to get our diagnoses right. The scientific aim is to diagnose mental illnesses correctly (not too broadly—yes, but also not too narrowly) and to diagnose when mental illnesses are *not* present.

I don't deny that there were some benefits with *DSM-III* and *DSM-IV*, but we should use science to correct and advance *DSM* revisions. Of course, politics is unavoidable, and practical considerations are relevant, but we shouldn't ignore legitimate scientific evidence. *DSM-IV* has been legitimately criticized for many reasons, and so will *DSM-5*. In my view, those criticisms are most legitimate when aimed at sacrificing scientific knowledge to professional expediency.

SOME ARGUE THAT EXPERTS are always biased in favor of expanding the realm of their diagnoses and further that scientific evidence is always too limited to stand on its own, hence the primacy of "pragmatic" factors. Readers will note by now that this latter comment betrays the standard belief system of the modern American: an unconscious postmodernism that is unduly suspicious of science and hardly respectful of the truth of anything.

It wasn't supposed to be this way. Somewhere along the line from *DSM-III* to *DSM-IV*, psychiatric leaders lost their way. In 1980, Robert Spitzer and Gerald Klerman and others who led the major revolution of *DSM-III* promised that science would have top priority in all revisions in the future. (Contrary to the claim that experts always want to expand their diagnoses of interest, the schizophrenia experts in *DSM-III* advocated *narrowing* that diagnosis; I, as a mood disorders and psychopharmacology researcher, have long advocated narrowing the MDD diagnosis and using fewer antidepressants and antipsychotics.) The fact that one had to pay attention to "pragmatic" considerations—

the beliefs of clinicians, the wishes of patients, our general ignorance about many scientific facts, the limitations of our treatments, the needs of insurance reimbursement—was accepted as a necessary evil.

But with the transition to *DSM-IV* in 1994, an important skepticism about science had seeped into the minds of nosologists; they concluded that science is, *and should be*, the least important factor in the *DSM* system; pragmatic, professional, economic, social considerations are *more* important. The process seems rather analogous to political gerrymandering: there are no "correct" borders, so let's fix things so we get elected more easily.

So, here's the sad secret of *DSM-IV*, revealed by its leaders: *Science matters least.*

THERE IS AN IMPORTANT consequence of this postmodernist evolution of *DSM*. Decades of biological research have been largely fruitless when applied to syndromes described in the third edition of the *DSM* or later. No biological markers have been defined for depression or bipolar disorder; no specific highly effective treatments have been identified; no genetic causes have been discovered.

Many blame the brain. The mind and brain are so complicated, it's argued, that it is just hard. It has taken two centuries for us to get this far; it will take many more to slog ahead slowly.

It may be that some of this blame should be shifted from the illness to us—those who claim to wish to understand these illnesses. We shouldn't be surprised that Nature doesn't follow a classification of diseases that we created almost completely on pragmatic grounds—for the purposes of insurance reimbursements, or deferral to the influence of social stigma in seeking to minimize psychiatric diagnosis, or the clinical belief systems of our colleagues or even the personal beliefs of nosologists. We shouldn't be surprised that these human, idiosyncratic motives are not reflected in biological markers, genetic tests, or drug efficacy.

A vicious circle of self-fulfilling prophecy has been created. Our pragmatic nosologists argue that our science is not sufficiently advanced to be the basis of our classification; thus, pragmatic judgments hold court. Yet those very pragmatic judgments create false diagnostic definitions that prevent our science from advancing enough to inform our nosologies.

THINK OF THE GREATEST scientific success in psychiatric history: neurosyphilis. Few are aware that about one percent of the European population circa 1900 was confined to mental asylums, many with neurosyphilis. In its early and middle stages, for decades at times, one cannot distinguish the mania, depression, and psychosis of neurosyphilis from what Kraepelin then called dementia praecox (DP) and manic-depression illness (MDI; see chapter 2). Yet by careful clinical description, psychiatrists were able to identify those with general paralysis of the insane (GPI)—an advanced stage of syphilis. Later, when syphilis tests were developed and the spirochete bacteria identified, studies of blood and brain in these patients showed that they had syphilis, in contrast to MDI and DP. If psychiatry had applied the *DSM*-pragmatic test in 1900, those GPI patients would have been mixed with the MDI and DP patients, and the later syphilis tests would have been all over the place; those biological studies would have been negative, neurosyphilis would not have been identified, and the astonishing success of the most effective psychotropic drug ever found—penicillin—would have remained unknown.

Some say there will never be another spirochete, that any other major biological causes of mental illness would have been found by now. Perhaps so. Or perhaps our failure to find major causes for an entity like MDD is because it is not a biologically valid entity. We are guaranteeing failure: if we continue to take this false pragmatic, postmodernist approach to *DSM* nosology, we will never know whether or not there is any other spirochete to be found. (Who knows: we might be surprised, just as happened with the discovery of the role of the bacterium *H. pylori* in peptic ulcer disease.)

Some believe our science will advance regardless of how we define diagnoses for insurance or other purposes. But *DSM-III* and *ICD-10* (*International Statistical Classification of Diseases and Related Health Problems*, 10th revision) have become much more than insurance documents. They are primary teaching tools in psychiatry training programs; often they have thus become, unfortunately, replacements for the actual study of psychopathology. They are also primary definitions used for research, ostensibly on the grounds of enhancing reliability. At least we are calling everything the same. Research grants are difficult to obtain, and studies difficult to publish, if *DSM-IV* or *ICD-10* criteria aren't used. These facts—the influence on both education and research—discourage researchers from testing and pushing the boundaries of *DSM* definitions. And even when such studies are conducted, as we have seen, the threshold for accepting changes to *DSM-IV* or *ICD-10* definitions has been set so high that few changes are made.

RELIABILITY (AGREEING ABOUT DIAGNOSTIC definitions) has been achieved, but it has not become, as once wished, a way station to validity (being correct about our diagnoses). Reliability is important, and useful, but it appears to have become an end in itself. Some of our nosologists celebrate, rather than bemoan, this evolution. With *DSM-III*, which originated with scientific impulses, the claim was made that reliability was the first step to validity. We would agree on our definitions and then we would test and change those definitions as the scientific data supported such changes. Now our definitions, such as MDD or hypomania, are so set in stone that better data than existed when they were initially defined are deemed insufficient to make further revisions.

For some, pragmatism is a necessary evil. Where the science is minimal or controversial, pragmatic judgments seem unavoidable. For others, pragmatism is better than science; it is to be celebrated as reflecting a profession's attempts to manipulate its diagnoses so as to counteract the baneful influences of other manipulators—such as the pharmaceutical industry, or ideological interest groups for or against specific diagnoses, or government agencies, or insurance bureaucrats, or the anti-psychiatry mob. Science is out of the picture, and, when it seeks to enter the picture, science is expelled as a pretender, a mask for "value" judgments, and a mere veneer for the motivations of those various other interest groups.

But if we accept that there is any reality to any mental illnesses, either as biological diseases in some cases or as identifiable social or psychological experiences in other cases, we have to stop treating psychiatric nosology this way.

WE COULD DO IT more scientifically, as have our colleagues in internal medicine. Or even, if we accept "pragmatism" as our ultimate belief-system, let's ask the pragmatic question: What are the results of "pragmatism" (in its postmodernist variety as enacted by the leadership of *DSM-IV*) versus science? Consider two contrasting timelines.

The first timeline, lasting fifty-six years:

1892: The "*DSM-I*" for internal medicine, *The Principles and Practice of Medicine*, by William Osler. The causes of pneumonia are unknown, treatments ineffective, outcomes mortal; but Osler describes the many features of pneumonias in careful, honest detail.

1948: Fifty-six years, and sixteen editions, later, and twenty-eight years after his death, the last version of Osler's textbook comes out the same year as the first randomized clinical trial of any drug, streptomycin for tuberculous pneumonia.

The second timeline, lasting sixty-one years to date:

1952: *DSM-I* for psychiatry, an administrative document for classifying hospitalizations.

1968: *DSM-II*, a slim document of neuroses and psychoses, largely ignored by practitioners and mostly used for insurance documentation.

1980: *DSM-III*, a doubling of diagnoses, the use of the word "disorder" to avoid saying what is disease and what is not, but the first attempt to base diagnoses on scientific research (as Osler had done).

1994: *DSM-IV*, some small changes based on science and many other changes based on "pragmatism."

2013: *DSM-5*

Which timeline had the greatest practical results?

It is clear: Osler's nosology was honest—and internal medicine jumped ahead in a burst of progress that in a century exceeded the prior two millennia. *DSM* nosology is dishonest—and psychiatry has stagnated for the past half century because of that dishonesty (and in the prior half century in the United States because of psychoanalytic speculation).

Without Osler's clinical detail and scientific rigor in diagnosis, the antibiotic revolution would not have been so easily applied to medical practice. Think about it: We have plenty of drugs in psychiatry, but we don't seem to know which patients should get them and which shouldn't. Some of us use them much, others infrequently, depending on our personal tastes. We boomerang between pharmaceutical libertinism and Puritanism.

Failure in biological and treatment studies may have been pre-ordained by our "pragmatic" nosology, designed to satisfy the personal

---

We have plenty of drugs in psychiatry, but we don't seem to know which patients should get them

---

views of its writers as to what is harmful, rather than to try to match up reasonably well to nature or to our knowledge of disease.

THE DICHOTOMY BETWEEN SCIENCE and pragmatism is false, as long as the science meets reasonable standards of quality.

The idea of pragmatism has an honorable genealogy. Invented by the nineteenth-century philosopher and mathematician Charles Sanders Peirce, pragmatism meant that we should judge the truth or falsity of our ideas not by some inherent quality but by their results in experience; a theory is tested in an experiment and the results of the experiment verify or falsify the theory. This is what Peirce—and later philosophers William James and John Dewey—meant by pragmatism.

Many psychiatrists, including the leadership of the *DSM-IV* revision, appear to set up pragmatism as an *alternative* to science—a meaningless distinction if we are talking about the term as used in the philosophies of Peirce, James, and Dewey. These philosophers argued that, where there is no or little science, pragmatic considerations are important, especially for legal purposes. But we should not let our "pragmatic" guesses outweigh science. Science should have priority. I say this fully knowing that science has its limits, that it can often be wrong—more: that it is always wrong to some extent. And that it can be misused, as in some of the pharmaceutically related research. I know that researchers have their pet ideas and blind spots; but so do nonresearchers. The beauty of science is that error is built into the process: in science, truth is corrected error, to use Peirce's phrase. Scientific work has no fear of being wrong, as long as one seeks to tell the truth as clearly and honestly as possible. The pragmatic approach involves a disregard for what is true—even when the research evidence provides reasonable evidence for what is true—at the expense of what we happen to think is useful or practical. This is pure utilitarianism, not pragmatism—a disregard for truth when one has only one goal, as Martin Luther King once said, "to get by." (Proponents of such "pragmatism" might want to listen to the moral denunciations of this attitude in King's sermons.)

Readers will avoid, I hope, the banal assumption that I must wish to rephrase all of *DSM* as biological disease. Quite the contrary. I think we need to do the honest scientific work of diagnostic description as seriously and as objectively as possible, so we can know and understand those conditions that are diseases, and those that are not. The "pragmatic" fear of made-up labels is valid, in many cases, but it is not valid when scientific evidence for disease is reasonably strong. We should accept both outcomes equally seriously, those where the evidence supports seeing psychological problems as diseases and those where it supports seeing those problems as nondiseases. Simply judging almost all conditions as "fads" and viewing everything as "labels" is simple, plausible, and wrong—easy to do from a reposed posture, but hardly advancing our knowledge. Psychiatry sits in the same place scientifically as medicine did at the end of the nineteenth century. If we are to experience the advances that medicine achieved, we would do well to study and follow the example of historical success. We should work vigorously to describe our psychiatric syndromes to the best of our current scientific ability, much as Osler did for medicine in his textbook. If that work is done objectively and honestly, then such definitions will promote and link to future advances in neuroscience and treatment, unlike our past "pragmatic" diagnoses. This scientific approach to medicine is exactly what Hippocrates supported against the "pragmatic" doctors who preceded him in the school of Cnidus, against which Hippocrates set up his school of Cos.

WHAT SHOULD WE BE pragmatic about? It seems to me that some justification exists for being pragmatic about treatment, as supported in a classic text of medical decision making but not about diagnosis. There the authors use a Bayesian pragmatic for diagnostic tests (as is standard in medicine) and for therapeutics. For instance, if one has a baseline likelihood that a clinical problem is present, based on the physical examination, then a positive test will increase that likelihood. Once the probability of that clinical problem really being present is high enough, then the doctor decides to give a treatment. If the treatment is highly toxic, the probability of a clinical problem would have to be higher (we would be more confident that the clinical problem exists) than if the treatment was more benign (we would have a lower threshold to treat). But applying such pragmatic notions to diagnostic criteria is an entirely different matter. In medicine, if one is going to use toxic chemotherapy, one wants a highly reliable diagnosis of cancer. If one is going to use aspirin, one doesn't need as reliable a definition of headache. But this pragmatic approach doesn't mean that we would alter the definitions of cancer so as to make it harder for clinicians to decide to treat it with chemotherapy. This is what *DSM-IV* nosologists tried to do. Cancer is cancer, and we need to be honest about it if we are to understand it better and get better treatments. The same holds for serious mental illnesses, like severe depression or bipolar disorder.

All these criticisms—of psychiatry, drugs, the pharmaceutical industry, diagnoses—are variations on postmodernism. They all fail because postmodernism is false. Bipolar disorder happens. Depression and mania are real experiences, often biological in cause, frequently needing medication. None of this detracts from our need to understand the experience of depression and mania better.

It's time to turn to the guides on the path, the ones whose thoughts have stood the test of time, the profound ones who speak to us quietly but truthfully.

III Guides

CHAPTER 10

Viktor Frankl
Learning to Suffer

IN THE MIDST of affluence, in contemporary America, we find mental starvation; the body is large and full, the mind dead.

There was a place and time where psychological death was natural, following upon physical desolation, a time when the deepest depths of human despair were tested, and where the existential approach to psychiatry received its most horrible experiment: Auschwitz. A psychiatrist was there to record and reflect on that experience, never knowing whether he would survive. Though all his family perished, Victor Frankl left the camps to tell us what that tragic event meant for human psychology.

Frankl noted that people had two initial phases on entering the camps: shock—followed by apathy, a dulling of all one's senses. For the rest of their stay, prisoners focused only on daily survival; higher thoughts, larger worries, dreams—all are put aside when all that matters is surviving. Where Freud famously saw most dreams as reflecting sex and aggression, Frankl found that the dreams of camp inmates were about "bread, cake, cigarettes, and a good warm bath in a tub." There was almost no sexual content to prisoners' dreams. The most common topic of conversation was food; sex, even in dirty jokes, rarely came up.

Freud thought sex was a primal human instinct. The camps were a deadly psychological experiment that proved otherwise: When facing the most profound limits of human existence, the most primal instinct was satisfying hunger for food and the deepest need was the mere fact of living.

LIFE IN A CONCENTRATION CAMP became, for Frankl, a harrowing intensification of the tragedy of life in general. All found themselves placed there, without cause, for an undetermined length of time, with no opportunity for pleasurable activity, with death an explicit daily possibility, and no means of escape. "The monotonous quality of life in the concentration camp led to the sensation of 'futurelessness.'" Inmates were forced to live as so many New Age gurus urge: they had no past and no future, so

---

The most horrible psychiatric outcome isn't suffering—it's apathy

---

they were forced to live in the present only. But in so doing, they plunged into a deep apathy, a "vegetative" existence whose only goal was to exist.

All knew that this was the worst outcome; Frankl wrote:

> The day would come when the apathetic inmates would simply lie on their bunks in the barracks, would refuse to rise for roll call or for assignment to a work squad, would not bother about mess call, and ceased going to the washroom. Once they had reached this state, neither reproaches nor threats could rouse them out of their apathy. Nothing frightened them any longer; punishments they accepted dully and indifferently, without seeming to feel them.

One Jewish camp doctor told Frankl that in his camp there was an expectation that they would be free by Christmas 1944; when the holiday came and went without freedom, there was "unprecedented mass mortality" in the following week. Prisoners stayed alive, literally, by force of will. When the will was gone, all was lost. Frankl concluded that the loss of a future guaranteed mental illness; to be healthy, one has to have a future.

Frankl identified something important from this tragic experience of the Holocaust: in the worst of existential circumstances, the most horrible psychiatric outcome isn't suffering—it's apathy. The worst scenario for the concentration camp inmate was not being anxious, or angry, or even depressed—it was becoming completely apathetic, giving up, not caring. Hence, Frankl concludes, we shouldn't fear suffering; we should fear not caring about whether or not we suffer.

CHAPTER 11

Rollo May and Elvin Semrad

I Am, We Are

ROLLO MAY TAUGHT a generation of psychologists to learn the importance of two words: "I am." Beyond all the intricacies of psychotherapy, the wish to understand, in a complex way, the complicated world of the mind—after all the ids, egos, superegos, Oedipus complexes, cognitions, and behaviors—May reminded us that at the bottom of it all is something much simpler and yet more profound: a human being, a person, an existence, me, you.

It is sad to say that perhaps the most important psychological fact—the basis for all psychology and psychiatry—is appreciated better by a child than by the average clinician: first and foremost, we are all human beings, and our most basic characteristic is that we exist. And we do so not in an abstract sense—of "Being" with a mystical capital B; not in a biological sense—of the living tissues of my body; but in a personal sense: I, me, Nassir Ghaemi, exist now, and so do you, reader, seated in your chair, glancing out the window, looking up at the clock. You exist *now*, reading me. I exist now, writing to you. ("This is no book; / Who touches this, touches a man; / (Is it night? Are we here alone?)" Walt Whitman, "So Long," verse 182).

This is the basic existential fact: that I am, you are, and each one of us exists in a special and unique and supremely important way that only each of us can comprehend individually. When a person goes to a psychotherapist or a psychiatrist, then, it is a poor clinician who doesn't

He discovered that the best protection against apathy in the concentration camps—the main means by which survival was promoted—was to suffer. Suffering prevented apathy. Those who suffered, survived; those who lost all ability to suffer, perished.

IN THE CAMPS, THE USUAL sources of meaning in life were foreclosed: no pleasure was available—no (consensual) sex, no (flavorful) food, no writing or reading, no traveling or vacationing, no gardening, no radio or music. There was no enjoyment or creativity to life. But there was suffering: Frankl found that suffering provided meaning to life, when pleasure was no longer allowed. Those who refused to suffer, who rejected the pain that was their only option to experiencing existence, had nothing left. Pleasure was denied them, and they rejected pain. That left nothing—their life became nothing, they became nothing, they died.

Frankl realized that the camps tore apart the veneer of the "cult of success." In the usual course of life, we tend to have the impression that meaning in life comes from achieving certain goals; we busily engage in the pursuit of those goals; we even sacrifice immensely—time, money, effort, relationships—for those goals. If we achieve those goals (fame, wealth, marriage, children), we believe we have attained meaning in our lives. If we fail, we believe meaning will have been lost, too. Here is Frankl's insight: In the camps, there was no option of success. *Everyone was forced to fail.* And yet, the experience of failure, the suffering engendered from it, also provided a meaning to one's life. So, too, in day-to-day life: we should strive, we should seek to achieve, but failure or success are each meaningful in their own ways. To fail is not meaningless, and there is benefit to be had from trying and not succeeding.

In the camps, if you failed to suffer, you died, literally, physically. In everyday life, if you fail to suffer, you die, metaphorically, psychologically. One case produces rigor mortis of the body, the other produces what Frankl called "psychic rigor mortis." The worst depression, he claimed, was not the melancholia of the suffering, tormented soul; it was the "melancholia anesthetica" of the apathetic, numb person who no longer cares.

THE OUTCOME MATTERS LESS than the process. In the camps, the outcome was preordained; there was no exit. Yet despair was not the only response. And the extreme example of the concentration camp is not too different, qualitatively, from typical life: there are many aspects of our lives that are not in our control, and indeed some that are likely so out of our control that they are in some sense preordained. (Perhaps Calvin was not so wrong.) So we have to face a dilemma that has something in common with (though obviously is not the same as) the camp prisoners: the problem of a destiny that we don't fully control. This doesn't mean we should not try to guide our circumstances toward our goals; but we need to be prepared to face exigencies we can't change. Destiny is "to be shaped where possible, and to be endured where necessary," said Frankl. Pleasure comes when we succeed; suffering when we fail. In each case, we must accept and even welcome both of those emotions, the wellsprings of our psychological lives—and keep living.

The experience of the camps taught Frankl that our concept of what is abnormal needs to be understood in the context of what is normal. *An abnormal reaction to an abnormal circumstance is normal*, he said; symptoms sometimes should be relabeled as accomplishments. This is especially the case with the experience of anxiety, in his view. To be somewhat anxious is normal; it's a sign of a healthy, even spiritual being. Biologists talk of the famous inverted U-curve of anxiety: Too little means you are in such a state of Zen-like calm that you will not react when an animal pounces on you from behind; too much means you are so agitated that you overreact and jump at the slightest perceived threat. In the middle is where we want to be. When someone experiences depression, the pathology can get worse and worse until one becomes completely apathetic; at that nadir, there is no anxiety. To be anxious, despite severe depression, is actually an accomplishment, a product of the personality strengths of the person who is depressed, fighting off the depression that would sap all one's will and take all anxiety with it. This is what Frankl means by seeing anxiety as an accomplishment rather than a symptom.

Most psychotherapies try to enhance our ability to achieve things or to enjoy life. Frankl hit upon an important aspect of existential psy-

chology that has been underappreciated; he made a new discovery: the goal of existential psychotherapy is to try to help us learn to suffer. The

---

The goal of existential psychotherapy is to try to help us learn to suffer

---

goal is to allow us to develop "a capacity for suffering as a possible and necessary task." It is an unfortunate, and fortunate, fact of existence that there is suffering. We must try to reduce needless evil and horrible suffering where possible, but we also need to learn, not only to accept, but to benefit from, whatever suffering remains. To suffer is to be human, not merely as a regrettable fact, but as a means toward a better end.

Frankl taught how to understand suffering. Another existential psychologist, Rollo May, would teach how to understand our encounters with each other as human beings. He is a second existential guide.

begin with this bedrock reality: the unique person who just entered the room. Only later might that person become a "patient," when a disease is identified, or a "client," when a life problem requires professional care, or—dare we clinicians ever have this courage—the person might just remain a "person" because she may turn out not to have any problem at all except the same ones that all human beings normally confront. She might even be patted on the back and sent home, reassured that she is a healthy person.

THIS IS NOT a strange concept. Many people act as if existential approaches to psychiatry are just completely at odds with medicine and science. All persons are patients to doctors. Some justify this usage in the sense that to be a "patient" means to "suffer" and the claim is that all those who seek help with doctors suffer in some way or another. But this is not true. Many of us feel quite fit, and then, on some routine visit, the doctor informs us that we have a disease; our suffering comes after the doctor visit, not before. (Is not hypertension the "silent killer"?)

It is the sign of the scientific physician, as the late Harvard psychiatrist Leston Havens informs us, that we are more often told we are healthy than ill. The doctor runs some tests; congratulations, on twenty-five tests you are normal; but on this one, you are sick. Even sickness is identified only in the context of larger health.

This is how medicine functions, when it is scientific. Health is a normative and common concept in medicine. It is usually the case; illness is the exception.

In psychiatry, matters are the reverse. No one goes to a psychiatrist or a psychotherapist without leaving the office pathologized; some "disorder" is labeled, and if not, some psychological complex or problem is identified. Existential psychotherapy is the only approach that begins with a premise of health, with the view that we are all normal human beings, and even our problems are the results of the same ("normal") challenges that all human beings must face as part of existence. Existential psychiatry, by beginning with the person rather than the patient, is in fact much more in line with scientific medicine than the pseudoscience of universal patienthood that afflicts psychiatry in all its other forms—biological, psychoanalytic, cognitive-behavioral, and so on. I say "scientific" medicine, because unscientific medicine is practiced—not just in psychiatry but also by many internists—whereby health is not respected and tests are excessively ordered, until something looks wrong enough to merit intervention, producing the corresponding monetary payment to the doctor, typically the ultimate goal of the whole process.

Rollo May was a psychologist who understood all this long before most American clinicians had any inkling of it. In the 1950s, May compiled and published the first translations of European writings on existentialism as applied to psychology and psychiatry. In the 1960s era and later into the 1980s, May became perhaps the most prominent homegrown existential psychologist in the United States. He was also trained in psychoanalysis, as modified by the American psychiatrist Harry Stack Sullivan (who, in turn, was an important influence on Leston Havens, who will be discussed in chapter 12), and May also used psychoanalytic concepts. He taught a healthy respect for the limits of psychoanalysis, though, a recognition that Freudian concepts worked where they worked and were misused elsewhere and an awareness of the power of existential concepts. I came to know of May's work more personally on developing a friendship with Ed Mendelowitz, a psychologist in Boston who studied with May in the latter part of May's career. In our discussions, Ed brought May to life, and, when reading his books, I heard the soul behind the words. I hear him speaking now, teaching us the fundamentals of the existential approach to psychology.

WHEN THE PERSON WHO is a clinician meets the person who is a potential patient or client, there is an *encounter*. This encounter happens between two human beings who meet on the same plane as human beings; they are persons with names, homes, backgrounds, ideals, values, wishes. Before any of the technical complexities of psychiatry can occur—before the doctor starts testing symptoms, or the psychoanalysts starts plumbing emotions—the two people must meet. This meeting may be simple. Leston Havens used to say that a good way to start it would be talk about the weather while walking down the hall from the waiting room to the office (in Boston especially, the inconstant weather is a suitable topic for such talk). After the weather discussion, the encounter might continue as the clinician tells the client a few things about herself: if asked, her education, experience, methods, goals. And the client tells the clinician, of course, about himself: his reasons for coming, goals, problems.

This may seem simple, and sometimes it is. Sometimes the encounter is bloodless, and it transitions seamlessly into the doctor-patient role. But sometimes it never transitions anywhere, and the whole relationship remains an encounter between two persons—and it gets bloody: That is existential psychotherapy.

Once the encounter gets started, it is not the task of the existential psychotherapist to attend to existential "themes." Existential therapy means getting rid of all themes, including existential ones. Meet the patient where she is. That's the first step. The therapist enters the circle of the patient's existence wherever the patient happens to be. (I use therapist and patient now to acknowledge the professional roles in my work as a psychiatrist, but I still wish readers to read those symbols as meaning "the person who is a therapist" and "the person who is a patient."). Usually, the patient comes with a problem; sometimes it's a relationship, sometimes a symptom, sometimes a sin. Whatever that problem is, May teaches that the existential therapist meets it first as a person's experience, not as pathology, nor in any other theoretical way.

The patient may have anxiety—*Angst*, better translated as anguish or dread. If so, May wants to know first whether it is normal anxiety or not. (He immediately avoids the presumption, which is typical of almost all nonexistential psychotherapy, that any symptom is abnormal.) Anxiety is a normal aspect of human existence; it is, Kierkegaard says, the "dizziness of freedom," the recognition that we have some choices to make in life. We always have choices (see chapter 16). Even choosing to live rather than to commit suicide is a daily choice we all make, consciously or unconsciously. We choose to do this or that, to study this or that, to work here or there, to marry him or her. Each choice is a step ahead toward our goals, but it is also a closing off of other roads. It is a birth, and a death. This is why we are anxious; anxiety arises, May says, at the borderline between being (what happens

---

Each choice is a step ahead toward our goals, but it is also a closing off of other roads

---

after we choose) and non-being (what we gave up). Being and non-being are in fact inseparable; one cannot be had without the other. They define each other. This is why life is enmeshed with death, why we cannot live fully until we accept death fully, why the greatest enemy of life is denial of death, why such denial is psychological murder.

So we experience dread, anguish, despair—all of us—not just prosaically in our daily choices but tragically in our awareness of death. Nothingness is the corollary of existence. So, May teaches, we can't really have an existential approach to psychology, we can't really appreciate human beings for who they are, we can't be humanistic, unless we have a tragic awareness of death. This kind of humanistic psychology is not the kind that uplifts, in any superficial sense. Once Ed Mendelowitz observed May at a lecture program in San Francisco, sharing the stage with other humanistic psychologists. A woman in the audience stood, after May made some comments along the lines I just provided, and said: Your view of humanism seems rather pessimistic; I prefer, the woman said, the ideas of Abraham Maslow (who emphasized authenticity and reaching one's potentials); I prefer to be joyous. May replied: I don't think I'm either pessimistic or optimistic; I'm realistic. I don't disparage your joy, he added, but I think true joy only arises from acknowledging our despair.

To get back to our prototype of existential psychotherapy, if the patient is anxious, then the therapist will try to see if the anxiety has to do with dread of life choices, or awareness of death. In either case, such anxiety is not a symptom, but, as Victor Frankl said, an accomplishment. It is to be applauded, not treated, and the goal of psychotherapy would be to help that patient acknowledge, bear, and put perspective on that anxiety (as Elvin Semrad, discussed later in this chapter, taught), so that he could then proceed with his life choices and with appreciating life in the context of death.

Anxiety as pathology, or neurosis (as is the label), happens when the patient can't tolerate such normal anxiety; the feeling of dread increases to a high level and paralyzes action and choice; the sense of despair about death reaches loud decibels, drowning out life itself, inviting suicide. The job of the psychotherapist then is to help lessen the severity of the anxiety symptoms, but even there, the goal is not zero—absence of anxiety and despair—but, to paraphrase Freud, the normal despair of the healthy human being.

Often, after the encounter has been underway for a while, the existential therapist will realize that the patient doesn't have *enough* anxiety; he doesn't suffer enough; he isn't tense about his choices; he is avoiding his limits and has no awareness of death. This is the apathy that Frankl noted in the concentration camps, the worst psychological outcome of human existence. We clinicians call this mental state "depression," not anxiety. It is a pure depression, unmixed with anxiety, completely apathetic, anhedonic—unable to experience pleasure—empty. *Melancholia* is the classic term, and it is apt—this is the black empty hole of nothingness that is the worst kind of depression. Here the existential therapist has discovered a disease, and the therapy moves from the encounter to the treatment, a biological one in this case: antidepressants or mood stabilizers (depending on whether the melancholia occurs in manic-depressive illness or not) or even electroconvulsive therapy. It is not at all incongruent for the existential psychotherapist to be a biological psychiatrist too; indeed, the philosopher and psychiatrist Karl Jaspers was exactly such a *biological existentialist*, someone who recognized and appreciated biology and science, as well as the limits of such science, and the freedom of existence beyond such biological limits (see chapter 14). Rollo May also repeatedly stated that existential psychology is completely consistent with science, not opposed to it.

SOMETIMES THE APATHY and absence of normal anxiety exist by themselves, without the melancholic depression of manic-depressive disease. In such cases, there is no medical diagnosis, but there are the twin existential problems: boredom and conformism. Sartre emphasized boredom as the key experience of this absence of normal *Angst*; a classic literary expression of it is Samuel Beckett's *Waiting for Godot*. Life is empty, meaningless; there is nothing to do, nowhere to go; we wait, not knowing what for, avoiding the only obvious destiny at the end of our waiting: death. This is the classic state of the teenage mind— no longer a child, not yet an adult, unable to take pleasure in life like a child, unable to understand death like an adult. Some of the sickest persons that an existential psychotherapist will see are adults who remain teenagers in their souls—bored and empty. They don't come to therapy with any specific symptom but rather with complaints about the consequence of their adult teenagehood: lack of meaning in life.

The existential therapist meets these patients where they are— on the problem of meaning in life—and, in so doing, the existential clinician has to practice philosophy. The problem of the patient is a problem that belongs to the field of philosophy, not psychology. Philosophers have important insights dating to millennia. It would be a narrow-minded clinician who would willfully ignore such wisdom. We cannot avoid philosophy, Frankl says, not because we therapists are attracted to it, but because patients bring philosophical problems to us. And yet, neither is the matter one of philosophy alone. The solution is not to ask our philosophy professors to become psychotherapists (which one group of psychologists and philosophers believes), nor to train psychologists in formal philosophy courses. Bertrand Russell and Alfred North Whitehead will not solve the problems of the masses of our psychologically dying citizens.

The consequence is a philosophical problem; that is why the existential clinician has to talk philosophy; but the cause is psychological— the absence of normal *Angst* about existence; that's why the existential clinician will use philosophy to return to the psychological roots of the problem.

BOREDOM IS ONE ASPECT of this existential condition: another aspect, which May emphasizes, is conformism. This is just as striking as boredom and much more dangerous. We again see it clearly in our teenagers: the ones who buy into the myth of popularity literally dress alike, from accessories to socks and footwear; they talk alike ("like, like, you know"); they act alike, walking in gaggles, haughty and disparaging toward others; they are cruel in groups, bullying sometimes even to the point of causing death in their victims. Teenage invincibility—the cliché captures the lack of awareness of limits, whether bodily or ethical or social. The result is a wish to be an unrecognizable part of the group. Go along. Get along. Social life—first and foremost.

To the extent that this is a phase in human development, one cannot begrudge it overmuch. But phases are supposed to run their course; they should end, and lead to something different, and often better. The teenage conformist ideally becomes the young adult, differentiating himself from his peers, getting to know the world in a personal and unique way, leading to the most important life decisions that can only be made authentically in accord with each person's unique tastes and abilities: choosing a profession, a spouse, raising children, maybe making a difference in the world.

But for some people, this type of teenagehood is not a phase but a finality: they become conformists, through and through, for the rest of their lives. May is explicit about this: by so doing, they have killed their Being. They are no longer in touch with their living core; their existence is defined by others, not themselves. To use Leston Havens's language, they are psychologically dead. The job of existential psychotherapists, should such conformists fall into their hands, is to resuscitate them, to bring them back to life psychologically. These are the toughest cases.

Death is the ultimate limit, the classic case of non-Being. And conformism is the most common means of avoiding coming to terms with non-Being. Says May: "Perhaps the most ubiquitous and ever-present form of the failure to confront non-being in our day is conformism, the tendency of the individual to let himself be absorbed in the sea of collective responses and attitudes . . . with the corresponding loss of his own awareness, potentialities, and whatever characterizes him as a unique and original being. "

MAY TEACHES THAT THE KEY to realizing the danger of conformism is to understand that the concept of being, the notion of our awareness of our existence, is equivalent to the concept of becoming, of achieving our potentialities. We are all born pluripotent, as the biologists would

---

We are all born pluripotent, as the biologists would say; we can go in any direction from childhood onward

---

say; we can go in any direction from childhood onward. We can select any profession, any spouse; we can move to any country, learn any language, take any religion. (The only thing we cannot change is our grandparents.) As each year passes, and we pass from childhood to teenagehood, to young adulthood, to middle age, and later—the alternative paths close ten by ten, two by two, one by one, until we become who we are: this person, me, at my age. We live often much longer, but the options in life are no longer there. We have arrived, psychologically, even though we have more life to live, biologically. Perhaps this is what George Orwell meant by his comment that at age 50, every man has the face he deserves.

To be is to become; being means having the possibility to be different things, to achieve different aspects of one's potential. The term "being" in English has a static connotation, May notes; we should probably use "becoming" instead to give a better sense of what the existentialists meant in their concept of individual existence—changing and fluid—as the ultimate reality. If we recognize this basic feature of each person's reality, then we can see that awareness of being is not about the present, or the past, but more properly, it is about the future: "The significant tense for human beings is thus the future—that is to say, the critical question is what I am pointing toward, what I will be in the immediate future."

So our conformist patient senses no meaning in life, because he ignores his being and nonbeing, he has no becoming, he has no future. Practitioners of existential psychiatry start with the absence of meaning, and, over time, show the patient how its root lies in conformism, and how the conformism is a failure to confront the realities of existence, of life and death. This is the course of existential psychotherapy in such persons, easier said than done, because it is only done through the encounter, the ongoing encounter, the increasingly bloody encounter as the patient gets to know more about the therapist, and the therapist more about the patient, and as they both together confront those unpleasant and tragic realities of human existence that we would all prefer were otherwise.

But if the problem is lack of meaning, the solution is to find meaning, and this is a psychological exploration of who one is, not an abstract philosophical discussion about what is.

To May, the solution happens when the patient has an "I am" experience. Here the problem is not that the patient doesn't have a sense of self, or of who she is, because of x, y, or z—fill in your favorite theory: psychoanalytic repression of unconscious wishes, cognitive distortions, the psychological effects of childhood trauma, poor parenting, personality traits, biochemical abnormalities. Those problems can cause abnormalities of self, and the existential clinician should look for them; but often they are assumed, rather than shown, and frequently, none exist, in which case the lack of sense of self is a primary existential problem itself: it grows out of a lack of connection with one's own being. In the course of the existential psychotherapy, in that setting, the therapist is seeking—through the encounter, through the hard work of empathy, of seeking to understand the feeling and meaning of the patient's experience—to nudge the patient toward the "I am" experience.

When it works out, the patient suddenly realizes that he exists—he is, here and now, in this world, and not only that: He *deserves* to be. He doesn't know why; he doesn't know how it happened; but he ended up alive, in this world, now, with these parents, in this culture, with this language, at this time. He may or may not like his parents; they may or may not value him; the same for his culture, religion, world. But here he is. He was meant to be here—now; and anyway he is here. Once he accepts it, and realizes that it is right for him to live, he can then go about deciding how he wants live: what he wants to do, how he wants to work, who he wants to love, what he wants to believe. But none of the rest happens unless he realizes and accepts the legitimacy of his existence. This is the "I am" experience; it is, as May says, the precondition for everything else: maybe he has psychoanalytic complexes, or too little serotonin so that he is introverted, or a biologically abnormal personality in some way; all that may be true, but none of it can be fixed until he first realizes that he deserves to be, until he accepts his being and becoming.

In a footnote, May describes how it may not be an accident how the Old Testament God names himself: "I am." Perhaps this awareness is the god within us, the recognition of our basic power of being, the reality of God as an existence.

There is much more to existential psychotherapy, but Rollo May is a clear and wise guide to its main features: encounter, awareness of being and becoming, normal anxiety, suffering, tragedy, the "I am" experience. Other guides, like Elvin Semrad, teach us how to move from "I am" to "We are."

IF MAY TEACHES ABOUT how anxiety can be normal, Elvin Semrad went further: He taught that psychosis could be normal.

We are all prone to make wrong judgments about others (and ourselves) based on inaccurate (or insufficient) information, which, some think, is not different in quality from the nature of delusions.

But we don't all have delusions, at least in the sense that delusions are supposed to mark out psychiatric illnesses. Some think that delusions involve problems in logic and reasoning; others that delusions grow out of abnormal perceptions (which are then normally reasoned). But perhaps there is another explanation (proposed by philosophers recently based on the ideas of Ludwig Wittgenstein): Wittgenstein held that we have "bedrock certainties" that are founded on having served us in acting in the world (these beliefs do not require rational or empirical justification). Go mow the lawn, we say, presuming that scissors will not be used.

Perhaps delusions occur because these very basic certainties, which happen before thoughts and sensations, steer us wrong. They are messed up in some way. If delusions are due to some basic existential abnormality, an inability to experience the world as it really is, then this might explain why patients can't be reasoned out of delusions; that's why they end up with psychiatrists.

We can't reduce knowledge to rationality or logic, nor can we reduce our understanding of delusions to cognition or sensation, nor even emotion (the usual alternative). Which leaves us with—not thinking, not feeling—just being: existence, with the clear therapeutic implication of an existential approach to treatment.

What does that mean?

I FIND MYSELF THINKING back to stories about the 1960s in Boston that I heard over and over again from my psychiatric teachers. At that time, the premier locus of psychiatric training and practice in Boston was Harvard's Massachusetts Mental Health Center, where the intellectual leader and residency director was Elvin Semrad. An aging, rotund Nebraskan, he had a gruffness to him, mixed with a Midwestern sensibility that he cultivated ("I'm just a hayseed from Nebraska"); he used this persona to make an impression, on patients and trainees, so that, along with a knack for the short memorable phrase, those who knew him came away with many "Semrad stories. " He wrote little and his reputation was passed along primarily based on an oral tradition of these stories. Here is a fictionalized amalgamation of the kind of interviews my supervisors used to describe to me that they had observed with Semrad, augmented by specific comments by him documented by his students.

Semrad ran a weekly case conference, where he interviewed patients; each week, psychiatry residents tried to pick their most difficult patients to test Semrad's interviewing skills. On one occasion, an enterprising resident brought a chronic, mute, unresponsive patient with schizophrenia from the "back wards" (meaning the parts of the hospital where those who are considered chronic and incurable are kept) of "Mass Mental." No one had succeeded in getting the patient to say more than a few words at a time, much less express any emotion. He was closed in the solitary cell of his insanity.

Semrad sat down on the podium, the residents below him in the audience. The patient was brought in, shuffling in from the side, guided on the elbow by the solicitous chief resident. The patient said nothing as he sat down, facing slightly away from Semrad. Semrad said nothing. They both sat awkwardly; Semrad finally broke the silence: "Thanks for coming, Jim." "Uh-huh," murmured the patient. Semrad sat silently some more, looking over the heads of the residents. Minutes passed. The patient shifted in his seat nervously; he glanced quickly at Semrad. Semrad peered at him, catching his eyes briefly: "Jim, it hurts." Jim shuffled some more; Semrad moved his weight from his left to his right. The audience was restless. "You loved her," he commented. "What?" said Jim. "You loved her—your mother—you loved her!" Semrad said, slapping his thigh lightly. Jim turned toward Semrad, then away, then back again and looked Semrad in the eyes: "You loved her," Semrad said more gently. Suddenly, Jim began to cry, the residents shocked at seeing any emotion in the patient. Semrad was unmoved: "You loved her." "I loved her," said Jim, sobbing. "But there was more," said Semrad ambiguously, hoping to bring out the ambivalence in all relationships. Jim pulled himself together a bit, sniffling some. "She was not easy," he said. "All mothers are like that," replied Semrad. And it went on, with the residents learning, for the first time, of a rather rich interpersonal life that had been previously locked away, how the patient had blamed himself for his mother's lack of attention to him; how when she was hospitalized for a psychotic illness, he had seen himself as somehow at fault; how all his life he had been the cause of all his misery. Semrad let him go on, looked at him sympathetically, commented on how he could not have possibly been that bad. After more back and forth, Semrad finally tied up the interview, and patted the patient's arm, as he got up: "Well, you seem like a fine fellow to me."

The patient was escorted away, and Semrad turned to his stunned audience.

"Tears never lie in a male." He paused, then added: "I've always thought that some of the things people suffer most from are the things they tell themselves that are not true." Semrad proved, repeatedly, that there was something to psychosis that was intuitive and nonverbal. Admitting that the patient was psychotic, Semrad would insist on his humanity: "And so often, when you get to know a patient, they lose

---

Some of the things people suffer most from are the things they tell themselves that are not true

---

their diagnosis, you know." All this led up to the classic Semradism: "No one is psychotic in my presence." And his interviews proved it—except Semrad thought it was simple: there was nothing importantly biological to psychosis, otherwise delusions would not be as amenable to his interviewing skill as they invariably were. Semrad failed to realize that there could be two truths here: psychosis could be biologically (and cognitively) based, yet it could also be existentially reachable.

Semrad proved clinically what philosophers seek to explain logically: delusions are not just about faulty cognitions or biological abnormalities (though they usually involve both)—they also involve something more deeply human, a basic existential fault, perhaps, reminding us that even in the most severely ill psychiatric patients, our clinical work involves—first and foremost—contacting the person beneath the patient, and saying hello.

If only we could do the same in our non-psychotic lives.

I NEVER KNEW SEMRAD personally; I wish I had. But I learned a lot about him, directly and indirectly, from his many Boston-area students. One of his closest disciples was Leston Havens, and I, like many others, had the good fortune of learning from Les for many years. If Semrad is the Marx of Boston existential psychiatry, Les Havens was its Lenin. He implemented and expanded and expounded upon those mysterious aphorisms of Semrad, and Les took it in his own direction. It is from Leston Havens (even though I was not formally trained in the Cambridge Hospital residency program, which he led for decades), more than any other person, that I have learned the most what psychiatry is all about.

CHAPTER 12

Leston Havens

Holding Opposed Ideas at Once

I TEACH THE PHILOSOPHY that we don't know, Leston Havens used to say. We don't know the truth; we don't know falsehood; we, in psychiatry and in life, are ignorant. As the old Argentine saying goes, experience is a comb you get when you're bald. Our knowledge is still-born. We are posthumously wise, too late for it to matter. And yet we live, and we live making decisions, all throughout our lives. And we want to know what the best decisions are. Semrad never wrote much. But, to answer those questions, we have the benefit of the written work of his close disciple, Leston Havens.

Les Havens was constantly faced with young, eager, intelligent residents coming to his Harvard residency program, wanting to know the truth about psychiatry. He was also constantly faced with (mostly) young patients, faced with one life dilemma or another, wanting guidance and wisdom. One man wanted to know if he should leave his wife, another whether he should stay. One woman wanted to learn how to love another, another how to stop loving too many others. One person needed to find out what to do with his life, another to see that he was doing too much. All took solace in this quiet unassuming psychotherapist, with his quizzical smile and friendly demeanor, who welcomed them into his old oak-lined dimly lit home office at 151 Brattle Street, near Harvard Square.

It is difficult to summarize the wisdom of Leston Havens, partly because that was his wisdom. He resisted firm belief systems, except perhaps his commitment to the freedom of each individual human being. It was difficult to tell where Les stood on any specific issue. If you brought up something with him, he would usually make some kind of comment that, subtly and indirectly, supported the opposite perspective. This was a psychotherapeutic technique, which he taught, called "counterassumptive" statements, as we'll discuss later in the chapter. But it had also become second nature to him, so that it pervaded all his conversation. Once, he said to me, "Nassir, most people kiss up and kick down; but you—you kick up and kiss down." And then he just looked at me; I couldn't tell if he meant it as a compliment or not. It felt like a compliment, because I knew Les valued someone standing up to the powers that be. But it also felt like a criticism, because I knew that Les was aware of some workplace conflicts that had arisen between me and others. Was he warning me? Or applauding me?

That was the paradox of Les Havens. He was doing both, as best I can tell—and that was his message. He often repeated a phrase he attributed to one of his favorite thinkers, Abraham Lincoln: Creativity meant "holding two apparently irreconcilable positions at once."

Hold your theories lightly, Les always said. This doesn't mean that no theory is true, so that you shouldn't bother committing yourself to any single one—not the postmodernist definition. Instead, he meant we can never be fully certain that a specific theory is true, and so, though we might be quite committed to it, we should leave an outlet, a way out, in case we're proven wrong—the approach taken by non-postmodernist but critically modern thinkers like the philosopher Karl Jaspers (see chapter 14), a man Havens greatly admired.

HAVENS STOOD FOR A *knowing ignorance*: that's what he meant by saying his philosophy was that we didn't know. He wanted us to know that we didn't know certain things we think we know, while at the same time being open to the fact that we can indeed know some things. (Can you hold two opposite thoughts in your head at the same time?)

Havens stood for ambivalence; since we couldn't be certain what was true, he was always searching for what might be true in the opposite perspective. In this approach, he drew a great deal on the American psychiatrist Harry Stack Sullivan, a man who had an active following in the Washington and Baltimore psychoanalytic communities from the 1930s to the 1950s. (Havens so often cited Sullivan that many had the mistaken impression that Havens had studied with Sullivan; they never met; Havens's knowledge came from his reading of Sullivan, especially the classic Sullivanian text, *The Psychiatric Interview.*) This approach led to some of Havens's favorite psychotherapeutic techniques. For instance, Sullivan taught "counterprojection." The patient "projects" his own thoughts onto the therapist or doctor; so in a paranoid patient (often with schizophrenia, the subject of Sullivan's work), one might be faced with thoughts that the doctor wants to harm the patient in some way. Food or medicine might be seen as poison. The patient might say: "All you doctors are on a power trip; I'm not taking that poison." Sullivan's approach would be to respond something like this: "Most doctors just want power; what a shame." A patient might blame his mother; to quote Sullivan, he'd respond: "Your mother was not an unmitigated blessing." Here is the classic ambivalent comment: Sullivan says that the mother was a blessing, in contrast to the patient's absolute dismissal of anything good; but, at the same time, Sullivan says that the blessing was mitigated, and thus in some ways not a blessing; and, the mitigation is stated as a double negative ("not unmitigated"), further burying the ambivalent message under indirect language.

You can imagine the reaction of patients: puzzlement. What did the doctor say? What did he mean? And with Leston Havens sitting in front of him, a patient would see that kindly quizzical smile, nonverbally sending the message: This is not a game; I really like you; and I'm here to help you.

LES WAS BIG on nonverbal communication. He wrote at length about the impact of how one sits, how one moves one's body, one's facial expressions—as ways of trying to connect and communicate with a patients. For instance, he emphasized the concept of "motor empathy" as a psychotherapeutic technique. Empathy is not only cognitive (thinking what the patient thinks) or verbal (repeating what the patient says) or emotional (feeling what the patient feels); it can be motor. When trying to empathize with a patient, Les would teach, start by sitting as the patient sits. If she crosses her legs, cross yours. If she looks down at a point in the ground, look at the same point; don't stare at her face as she looks away from you. I've been amazed over and over again that when I use this motor empathy technique, I find patients naturally looking up and looking me in the face—and then we can talk.

These methods are all about connecting with the patient and also about speaking up for more than one side of an issue. It's hard to connect with another human being, and it's easy to fall into one way of thinking, to take one dogma as the truth. We all have our dogmas; it's easy to say that dogmas are bad, but we all live with many dogmas that we would kill for. Jaspers called them "life-sustaining lies"; take away someone's life-sustaining lie, and they will despise you. That's what Havens did in psychotherapy, it seems to me: very gradually and with exquisite attention to developing a strong human connection with the patient, Les would strip away the life-sustaining lies in that person's life that were, in fact, strangling his or her life. At the end of therapy, the person was free of the lies, and now free to be whoever he or she really could be.

Havens once gave an example of this holding-opposite-ideas approach in what he called the "classic male dilemma: Should he stay with his wife or leave? I took both sides. The improvement was: He slowed it all down." Havens didn't know the answer, but he wanted to make sure his patient looked at all sides of the question. So whatever direction the patient went, Havens would go in reverse. If the patient turned to follow him, then Havens would speak in favor of the patient's original thoughts. There's no correct answer, but there is a correct approach: paying attention to all sides of the question.

That was the goal of psychotherapy, in Havens's view: *personal liberation*. He practiced psychotherapy like a revolutionary liberation movement. He transferred the concepts of democratic thinking from politics to psychotherapy. Havens was a political psychiatrist, in a unique way that has never been previously implemented. Hence his frequent citation of thinkers like Lincoln or the Founding Fathers or Gladstone or Churchill in explaining his approach to psychotherapy. He saw therapy as involving "successive acts of liberation, not moving speeches or penetrating insights."

LES BELIEVED THAT a major source of the huge problem of stigma, of discriminatory attitudes about mental illness, was mental health clinicians. Clinicians tend to blame everyone else: society, the media, anyone else but themselves. They imagine they don't have stigmatizing attitudes merely because this is their work; in fact, they constantly stigmatize their patients. (Some would say our language is stigmatizing, though I'm not a fan of changing a word, like "clients" for "patients," unless one changes one's attitudes first.).

Les said that clinicians stigmatize patients from the start: they treat them as an "other" and pretend to know them when they don't; when patients go to the medical doctor, he lays hands right on their bodies. He gets to know them, physically. Mental health clinicians don't touch our patients—hence the distance, physically and psychologically. How can they get to know this person in front of them?

Right from the start, immediately, Havens emphasized that we need to give the patient "a sense of at homeness." Ending stigma begins at home, in the clinician's home, in his office.

We next have to realize that a major assumption in medical work is absent in psychiatric work. When the patient goes to his internist, he is assumed to be "cooperative and reliable." When he goes to his mental health clinician, "by definition," he is perceived as uncooperative and unreliable: something is off in his relationship with others. He might be afraid of clinicians and their diagnoses. Whatever the reason, the psychiatric patient is ambivalent: he wants help but he can't easily cooperate in the process.

Hence, before any psychotherapeutic work in the service of personal liberation could begin, Havens realized that a person's life-sustaining lies would be so dearly held that they would never be given up until the patient could fully trust the therapist. The first and primary goal of psychotherapy was to establish a "safe place" (the title of one of his books) for the patient to be able to reveal and discuss his deepest thoughts and fears and wishes. This creation of a safe place is incredibly hard work. In fact, it might be correct to say that, in Havens's approach, almost all the work of psychotherapy goes into creating that safe place.

It's not the work of the therapist to tell the patient what to do, or to figure out what is the right answer; the patient will find the right

---

The goal of empathy is enough safety to begin to find out the painful truth

---

answer after all the deceptions and self-deceptions and clearly wrong answers are revealed for what they are.

The work of creating a safe place is the work of making a setting where that clearing-away work can be done, as safely and as painlessly as possible, knowing all the while that it is dangerous and painful work, which could easily make a patient more symptomatic and even lead to psychiatric hospitalization, or even death by suicide.

Creating the safe place involved first and foremost, and in the end, empathy. The work of the therapist was to identify with the patient and to help the patient identify with the therapist, so that after a while, there was no longer therapist and patient, but two human beings struggling together with human problems. This is existential psychotherapy: the transformation of the clinician-patient dyad into a human-human dyad.

Eventually, by the end of the therapy, both would be changed—the therapist and the patient. Let me emphasize, in contrast to the usual postmodernist interpretations of empathy, that the goal of empathy is not empathy per se but rather enough safety to begin to find out the painful truth. Havens said that it was about two subjectivities meeting and moving in the direction of objectivity.

I'VE DISCUSSED SOME SPECIFIC techniques, like motor empathy, that Havens used in this process. Here are some comments from his writings that give a flavor of what he meant by this empathic process overall: "Every treatment is in part a treatment of the doctor, if only of his pretenses" and "We need someone enough like us to share our experience, and different enough to have a separate perspective."

Empathy is a step, in fact many steps and leaps and bounds, but it is not the destination. Freedom is the goal. To get there, one has to stop empathizing. Empathy allows one to understand the patient and get the patient to allow the work to begin. But then the work has to happen. That's what Havens meant by having a different perspective. Empathy doesn't mean agreeing with the patient; it means agreeing enough so that the patient can hear your disagreement. Here we see the influence of Semrad—his formula of psychotherapy being about helping the patient acknowledge, bear, and *put perspective* on his emotions.

One of the key things you have to learn in psychiatric residency, Havens used to say, was to hang up the phone. Hang up the phone on your patients. Don't always be available; set limits; stop talking; get them to stop talking. Empathy doesn't mean being a pushover; you have to also push back, but only after you've gained the patient's trust.

ANOTHER KEY HAVENESQUE CONCEPT is the notion that everything is a fiction until proven a fact. Havens struggled with how his ideas, especially the Sullivanian counterassumptive approach, could give the impression of disingenuousness. After all, the therapist doesn't *really* agree with a schizophrenic patient's paranoid delusions about the FBI, but Havens would try to agree with the patient as a matter of technique, and he at least would avoid overt disagreement at all costs. If you believe telling the truth, under all circumstances, is a virtue, then Havens's approach to psychotherapy is a vice. Havens was aware of this problem, and he managed it with his other idea of holding your theories lightly. One never knows anything absolutely definitively, and so, it is not technically disingenuous to agree with even the most outlandish idea, even if one thinks it highly improbable.

A medical student once asked Havens why it is that so many psychotic patients say they hear the voice of God.

Havens paused, moved toward the student, looked him in the eye, and said solemnly: "You don't think God would speak to just anyone, do you?"

IMAGINE CONDUCTING A PSYCHIATRIC interview, or psychotherapy session, without ever asking a question. This is what Les Havens sought to do. Make comments; no questions: That was his ideal.

It's incredible once you try. One develops a totally new way of talking with someone else. (I also recommend this technique to single persons on dates.) Most of us talk to each other as if life was a question-and-answer session. This is especially the case in the medical and clinical tradition. I find that young psychotherapists are often nervous because they don't know what the "answers" are; I try to put them at ease by teaching Havens's method of avoiding questions so that the problem of answers never arises.

You can't get at the truth with questions, Havens believed; and therapists have no answers to provide anyway. When you ask a question, you immediately put the patient on the defensive. He thinks to himself: what's the right answer? What does he want me to say? Should I say what he wants to hear? Asking a question is like a frontal assault in military strategy: it should be employed rarely and only when there is overwhelming force. Making comments are like flanking movements in battle: first you test the right side, then you test the left, trying to see whether you can find a place to enter.

This approach, which Havens called "soundings," is something he analogized to "perscussion," the medical method used to examine the body (now less used since x-rays and other imaging have become common). The doctor would tap his fingers on the patient's belly or chest or back, knowing where the organs are supposed to be (producing a dull sound), knowing where there should be nothing (producing a hollow sound). The doctor doesn't ask the patient if his liver is large or if his lungs are full of fluid; he sounds things out physically.

Similarly Havens thought we should stop asking patients what is going on with them and start to sound things out psychologically. This method can be exemplified with the method of assessing suicidal thoughts. The usual questioning method is easily distorted by the patient's awareness of what the doctor wants to know and with the fact that patients generally are smart enough to know that there are consequences to how they answer (including involuntary hospitalization) that they may or may not want to avoid. So the simple method is asking: "Do you have thoughts of wanting to hurt yourself?" or "Do you have thoughts of not wanting to be alive?" With these simple questions, patients know what to say, depending on what they want to get out of what they say. This is the psychiatric equivalent of Pickett's Charge, straight at the center of the Union line in Gettysburg. It's hard to succeed if the enemy wants to resist.

Here is the soundings approach of making comments; I've put my thoughts as the interviewer in italics (these are my thoughts, not Havens's):

I think this patient has some suicidal thoughts, but I'm not sure how serious they are, and I know she is reluctant to tell me partly because she doesn't want to end up in the hospital. I decide to start by underestimating her suicidality. I'm looking at the ground, not at the patient, because she is looking out the window, and I want to appear as unthreatening as possible. I punctuate my statement with many hems and haws, to accentuate the air of uncertainty. "I suppose, hem, that you never, uh, have any thoughts, mmmm, of not wanting to be alive." (The words "I suppose" or " I imagine" were a staple of Havens's talk.)

The patient looks right at my face. "Well, you can't ever say never."

Now I realize she's open to admitting something, but I need to remain light in touch. I look at her briefly, then back at the ground. "Well, I guess we all sometimes have those kinds of thoughts, but maybe it hasn't happened to you recently."

Now she has to commit. Either it has happened recently or it hasn't. She looks away again. "I don't know; it's hard to say."

She's not going to make it easy. "Well, I imagine it might have happened recently, and you might not remember, or maybe you'd be afraid to mention it to me."

She's looking at the ground now where I'm looking. "Yeah, maybe."

I'll take that as a yes, and conclude that she has recent suicidal thoughts, and that's all I'm going to get out of her now. I just want to make sure she doesn't have immediate serious thoughts. Now I look her straight in the face. "You might even want to kill yourself right now, for all I know!" *I smile, to give the impression that maybe it's a joke, that I'm not so serious that if she says yes, I'm immediately going to call security to put her in the hospital.*

She laughs: "Are you kidding, doc? If I was, I wouldn't tell you anyway."

I laugh: "I know that. And if you were, I'd just guess anyway, and do what I needed to do."

Notice how much of the communication was nonverbal.

HAVENS'S AMBIVALENCE, HIS BELIEF in holding opposing theories in your head at the same time, is best expressed, I think, outside of his psychotherapeutic methods and is seen best in his conceptual work on the nature of mental illness. His classic oeuvre is his 1973 *Approaches to the Mind,* the best single book, in my opinion, on psychiatry in the modern era.

I have a deep fear about Leston Havens: Most people don't know about him, and those who do know him, misunderstand him. He seems to have had the worst outcome: either being unknown or distorted. I may be wrong in my own interpretation, but here it is; I can say I've expressed these ideas to him directly, and he agreed with me, although, as I've said, it was always hard to know if Les fully agreed with you on anything or not.

Havens taught for about thirty years at Cambridge Hospital, most as director of its psychiatric residency. Literally hundreds of psychiatrists interacted with him directly for three years or more on multiple occasions; they sat in hours of individual or group supervision with him discussing many cases. They heard him give case conferences and lectures over and over again. And I would wager that almost none of them would know that Havens's first psychiatric publications from the 1950s, when he was just starting his career, had to do with biological treatments: amphetamines and electroconvulsive therapy. He once told me this fact with great relish, as if it was a secret just between the two of us. One might excuse his many students; he never hid his biological origins, but he never emphasized them either.

He and I had a bond on this matter because I was the "token" biological psychiatrist at Cambridge Hospital in the early 2000s. I had never trained there, instead doing most of my training at the very biologically oriented Massachusetts General Hospital (MGH) department of psychiatry and at the very research-oriented McLean Hospital (all affiliates of Harvard Medical School, like Cambridge). Cambridge, in contrast, was the "touchy-feely" psychosocially oriented Harvard program; the hospital was a small community institution, founded in the 1960s, and it always had a strong social, even socialist, orientation. Patients didn't pay for care; the city of Cambridge did; all the poor and huddled masses were welcome. They received much empathic listening, à la Semrad, and few drugs; there was hardly any research.

At the center of it all stood Havens, the pied piper of this merry, radical, left-wing bastion of Harvard psychiatry.

I had gotten to know Havens and Cambridge when I was a visiting medical student from Virginia. I had never seen anyone interview patients so wisely and humanely. His charisma was remarkable. When trying to decide between the big three Harvard psychiatric residencies, I was tortured. MGH seemed too single- and simple-minded for my taste; McLean was broad and solid and promised to expose me to all different approaches to psychiatry; but then there was Cambridge, which meant Havens, with the promise of a special wisdom. My mind told me to go to McLean; my heart said Cambridge.

I interviewed with Havens, a life-changing hour in which what I remember best is that benign, solicitous face. "You want to learn about research," he said near the end. "You should go to McLean. We don't do any research here." With that, he made the decision for me. I went to McLean, and later MGH, and still later when I decided to leave the MGH faculty for professional reasons, after having begun to establish myself as a researcher in psychopharmacology, I thought once more of my first love, Cambridge. I called Les, and I interviewed again, this time for a faculty position, and this time the hospital leaders offered me a job, asking me to start research at Cambridge in psychopharmacology. I did what I could for five years, but the best outcome of those years, from my perspective, was the weekly supervision I received from Les, supervision about anything and everything, mostly about my work. He encouraged and helped me as I wrote my first book, *The Concepts of Psychiatry,* in particular.

All this is to say that Les supported me as the token biologically oriented psychopharmacologist at an institution that was suspicious of such thinking. And the reason was that Les himself had been a biologically oriented psychopharmacologist. And he still valued biology and psychopharmacology in psychiatry, far more than most of his students and followers.

This fact became clear for me one night when I invited David Healy to speak to the monthly History of Psychiatry group organized by Paul Roazen (see next chapter) at the Harvard Faculty Club. Les, who was a regular attendee, listened with about two dozen others as Healy presented his ideas about the history of psychopharmacology, about how many of the past antipsychotics were actually harmful and neurotoxic, about how antidepressants caused suicidality, and how the pharmaceutical industry had influenced the profession to overestimate the benefits of medications. I knew Roazen, who was a good friend of Havens, agreed with Healy on most of these matters; I also agreed with him on some of those points. But, to everyone's surprise in the mostly sympathetic audience, Les Havens was getting increasingly red in the face; by the end of the lecture, this amiable, mild-mannered man lost his temper. He stood up and raised his voice: "This is all wrong," he exclaimed. "How can you say such things!?" I don't recall any specific criticism, but I do recall that Les was generally critical, thinking that Healy incorrectly undervalued medications.

I had driven Les to the event, and he got up to leave. I stood up to leave with him. On the way to his house, he was still fuming. He didn't say anything; he didn't need to say anything more.

THE PARADOX OF LESTON HAVENS is the paradox of freedom, his ultimate goal for his patients. The holding of opposite thoughts together was the constant theme, so much so that it seemed to be what he meant by freedom. He repeats, over and over in his writings, variations on this idea: "I must be as free and as compliant as I dare." In another place, he writes: "Psychic health requires both freedom and compliance—the ability to connect and disconnect, to connect with others and to leave and protect oneself from others." Havens compared

> **Psychic health requires the ability to connect and disconnect, to connect with others and to leave and protect oneself from others**

this to nutrition, which involves both eating and not eating. It is so easy to get into dogmatisms: some people think that psychotherapy should be all about "authenticity," be who you are, follow your dream, be a nonconformist, and the like. It's easy to repeat these graduation commencement platitudes that are destroyed by the realities of life.

In psychotherapy, platitudes go nowhere.

Havens realized that we should dream and not conform, but sometimes, our dreams are impossible; sometimes we should conform.

He asked: "How do you give someone freedom?" Freedom can't be given; it can only be taken away. He said the goal of therapy was "to be neither possessor nor possessed." Thus: "Treatment is less a curing than a learning to live."

This whole process is not intellectual, as in most psychotherapies, which are based on the psychoanalytic tradition. Freud's followers thought they could capture the truth in some formulae and pass those truths along to patients in the form of "insights." Havens, a psychoanalyst who had grown into existential thinking, realized that the intellect was feeble, and that change wasn't even emotional, and certainly not something more abstract ("spiritual"); his metaphors for psychotherapeutic change, going back to his biological roots, were almost physical: "As time passes, [the] task seems to me more and more a matter of growing things, of movements and feelings, and less a matter of words and ideas—in which my own effort, too, may be imprisoned." Or: "I judge the success of psychotherapy in two ways. Does the patient's appearance change? Does he get new friends?"

IN OTHER WORDS, Leston Havens tried to get at the "person inside the patient." He tried to get at the person's existence, in addition to, or instead of, his diagnoses and symptoms. A common mistake among those attracted to his humanistic approach is that the words "in addition to" are always replaced by "instead of." Neither approach can be presumed. Sometimes patients have diseases, and these are diseases of the body, and Havens would be the first to argue that if we have effective drugs, they should be given for such diseases. Sometimes, though, people don't have diseases of the body but problems of living. In those cases, the psychiatric work consists of getting to know the person's existence, who she is as a human being, not her symptoms or made-up diagnostic labels. Critics of biological psychiatry are dogmatists who always take the latter approach. Simplistic practitioners of *DSM*-slap-dash psychiatry are dogmatists who always take the former approach. Les Havens asks you to hold both ideas in your mind at the same time and realize that sometimes there is a place for one and sometimes for the other. (And it is not up to you the clinician to choose eclectically, "individualizing the treatment" as you wish; science tells us which is which.)

Havens highly identified himself with his medical heritage. He was always comparing and contrasting the work of the psychiatric clinician with that of the general physician—how they were similar and how they differed were equally important to Havens. I mentioned earlier that Havens pointed out that psychiatric work has the major disadvantage of not being able to examine the body, as in general medicine. Havens once suggested that the work of getting to know the patient's existence is the closest substitute. The patient's existence is like the body; it is what we can feel and touch and know in a way that goes beyond what the patient says, even with years and years of talking in psychotherapy. It's not all about what the patient says; what matters also is how the patient looks and acts and moves and feels; what she values and does and imagines and hallucinates.

Havens always emphasized the relationship between doctor and patient, the therapeutic alliance; he was convinced that this relationship was the key treatment in psychotherapy, not any specific theory or idea about how to do psychotherapy, not any specific insights on the part of patient or doctor, not anything anyone said. It was the relationship itself that mattered most. But Havens took this view, commonly assented to by many clinicians, and he made it more profound; he thought the relationship was not an end in itself, as many presume, but a way station to the patient's freedom, a freedom that could not be proscribed or prescribed or even defined.

Toward the end of his life, Havens was more and more concerned with the concept of the self; he wanted to know what it meant. It seems to me that he was trying to explain the end result of psychotherapy. This existence is the person; it's the self. Person and self and existence are all one thing in the end. Psychotherapy involves the person becoming free to become himself. To paraphrase Nietzsche, one becomes who one is.

HAVENS ONCE SUMMARIZED HOW you get to this goal of getting to the person inside the patient. He said there were five aspects: First, you struggle with the patient—you conflict as you get to know each other. Then, you develop a kind of "comradeship," a feeling of fellowship, an at-homeness has been established. You then simply are with each other, being together, until you have an "Aha experience," like May's concept of the encounter. Something happens, and you and the patient both realize something that you didn't previously. Gradually, as you keep meeting and being with each other, you both change. The patient becomes new-patient; the doctor becomes new-doctor. Both persons in the treatment change. This is quite important and unique to Havens compared with so much of the dull psychotherapy that happens these days. If the clinician doesn't change, then the therapy can't be successful. Every treatment is in part a treatment of the therapist. Finally, Havens draws on Martin Buber to say that clinicians need to "imagine the real"; they need to go beyond what the patient herself might say or believe and "speak for a person's life." If the patient doesn't dare to dream, the clinician must dream for her. The clinician must lead the patient. In the end, after all the work of getting to know each other and changing gradually together, the clinician has to point the way to a new existence, an existence that the patient and clinician have imagined together.

At the end of psychotherapy, if it all has worked out as Havens would want, the patient is let go, finally now free, with a direction pointed out by the therapist, a new path to take where one's dreams wait along the way. The work of the psychotherapist is finished: Only the patient can actually walk that path.

THE OVERWHELMING IMPRESSION ONE got from Leston Havens, as a teacher or a therapist, was the expression of hope and courage. Les was always encouraging you to do what you think you can do, to do more, to do what others haven't done. He gave you the courage you didn't have. He always stood for hope, tempered by realism, but hope nonetheless. "Much that patients tell us is little more than a test of our courage," he said.

He definitely had a parental instinct, a sense of nurturing others that felt quite maternal in fact. He often analogized the task of the therapist to the "the curious mixture of letting alone and occasionally nudging," much like the attitude parents have toward their children. It's a kind of silent prayerfulness, where you have a good idea of what is the right thing to do, but you can't just say it, and you can't make it happen. You can only watch and hope and nudge your child (or patient) along as best you can.

This was probably what lay behind one of his favorite poems, Richard Wilbur's "The Writer," where a father watches his daughter writing in the attic, and a bird flies in the room and tries to fly back out but hits the partially open window. Father and daughter silently watch and pray, as the bruised and battered bird tries to find its way out the open window slit:

. . . how our spirits
Rose when, suddenly sure,

It lifted off from a chair-back,
Beating a smooth course for the right window

IN WHAT I BELIEVE was Les's last public lecture before gradual dementia took away his phenomenal oratorical abilities, he gave a talk at Cambridge Hospital about a fifty-year view of psychiatry, denoting his career. In that lecture, his final theme was: What is your dream? He asked that question repeatedly; he said that our work in psychiatry involved getting patients to the point that they could become aware enough to answer that question.

We all have dreams, Havens said, paraphrasing May Sarton: Who would wash the dishes without a wild vision of the future? And yet we quash our dreams prematurely, or we give them up in childhood, the only stage in life where we naively dream freely. Outside childhood, the only other free dreamers are people with manic episodes.

Les and I wrote about mania in 2005, and Les was clear that he thought one could, and should, empathize with mania in someone with bipolar disorder. Les saw clearly what it took me more years to appreciate: there are many positive aspects to mania and depression that we should celebrate, not simply treat away.

The psychoanalytic tradition had ignored mania, or just seen it as a superficial flight from depression. Les thought mania was profound on its own grounds, because it exemplified the essential trait of having dreams, of having wild visions of the future, without which we can never achieve great things. He said we should empathize with mania because we normal persons also have manic-like ideas.

He liked to use the example of New Year's Eve celebrations. In some ways, what a foolish idea such celebrations are: Why should the events of the next year be any better than those of every year past? And yet,

---

Who would wash the dishes without a wild vision of the future?

---

we celebrate the New Year, each year, with revived hopes and renewed ambitions. Omar Khayyam realized how solemn each new year truly is:

The New Year reviving old Desires,
The thoughtful Soul to Solitude retires,
Where the White Hand of Moses on the bough
Puts out, and Jesus from the ground suspires.

The Rubaiyat of Omar Khayyam, verse 4

LES HAD GREAT AMBITIONS for himself, though he hid them behind a mask of modesty. He had his own grandiosities. "I wanted to kill Hitler!" he once told me passionately and unironically, explaining why he had enlisted in World War II. He came across to most people as unassuming, almost too humble; I am convinced it was an unnatural exercise of great effort, an attempt to control his natural ambitions. Readers can see that I think his gifts matched his ambitions, and those who knew him knew they were in the presence of some kind of greatness.

What has eluded his students is exactly what that greatness was, somewhat as happened with Semrad.

I've concluded that a central feature of Havens's teaching is the willingness to hold, even search for, opposing ideas at the same time—the touchstone of his concept of freedom. One of Havens's close personal friends, the historian of psychoanalysis Paul Roazen, was another guide who shared this way of thinking. Roazen taught how to think honestly, in the face of the most popular ideas, and see what was bad in what was good. To him we now turn, as our next guide.

CHAPTER 13

Paul Roazen

Being Honest about the Past

A POLITICAL SCIENTIST WHO became convinced of the importance of psychoanalysis for all intellectual work, Paul Roazen was a central chronicler of the history of psychoanalysis. During decades of work that ended in his death in 2005, he saw the history of psychiatry, not as merely an academic matter, but as a means of improving the practice of psychiatry itself.

As a young Harvard graduate student in political science in the 1960s, Paul Roazen took an interest in how psychoanalysis might relate to political theory. Others had conceived of this connection in the past (like those at the neo-Marxist Frankfurt School) but Roazen's interest was piqued not by Freud's theories, but rather by the living Freudians he saw around him. In his hometown of Boston, Roazen came across a bevy of middle-aged and aging Viennese and Germans with their thick accents and old-fashioned clothes, and he realized that he could learn about psychoanalysis from these people.

Soon Roazen was tracking down and interviewing every single psychoanalyst he could find who had any relation to Freud. From them he heard stories about their patients and then he turned to tracking down living patients of Freud and the early Freudians.

Roazen the political scientist became Roazen the oral historian. He still wanted to link psychoanalysis and political theory, but he didn't want to base his understanding of psychoanalysis solely on reading Freudian works. He wanted to learn from the Freudians themselves.

Learning entailed not only conducting his interviews but also attending clinical case conferences at the Boston teaching hospitals. Roazen began this practice by attending the weekly conferences of the Massachusetts Mental Health Center, then the most prestigious Harvard institution, where Elvin Semrad taught. One of Semrad's top lieutenants and the focus of the previous chapter, Leston Havens, would spend the next four decades in weekly conversations with Roazen about all aspects of psychiatry and psychoanalysis.

Even after moving to Toronto (where he spent the bulk of his career as a professor at the University of York for much of the 1970s and 1980s), Roazen remained highly connected to his clinical friends and never gave up his attempts to understand psychoanalysis from the clinical side, not just from theory.

I MET PAUL IN the late 1990s in Cambridge, Massachusetts; he had since retired and returned to the city of his birth. Freed from all academic responsibilities, he had turned to his loves of reading, writing, and lecturing. In fact, in the decade after his retirement, he published more books than in the previous two decades of his most active academic work. I met him at the psychiatric grand rounds of Cambridge Hospital, which he attended weekly; Leston Havens introduced us, and, following that meeting, Paul added me to his list of regular lunch partners.

By the time I left the Boston area in May 2005 to move to Atlanta, Paul and I had become close, and we had planned to meet again when I returned over Thanksgiving. It didn't happen. In early November 2005, Paul died suddenly at age 67.

In the intervening years, I have turned to reading more of his works and, perhaps in working out my own grief, have come to the conclusion that this esteemed historian of psychoanalysis himself deserves a record of the history of his own journey, a distillation of his ideas and ways of thinking, a passing on to future generations of his great effort to understand this complex discipline, psychiatry, so as to help us—the clinicians—to be better at what we do.

IN A WAY, PAUL Roazen practiced history as gossip; his oral history was formalized gossip. Indeed, one of his books, *How Freud Worked: First-hand Accounts of Patients*, involved detailed description of how Freud exactly practiced psychoanalysis based on Paul's interviews with the last living former patients of Freud in the 1960s and 1970s. This invaluable historical record puts the lie to almost all the standard teachings of psychoanalytic method, at least in the hands of its originator. One review of the book was titled "Psychogossip." Paul loved to gossip, about almost everything, including what his Cambridge neighbors thought about the garbage practices of certain Harvard faculty. Being an oral historian was true to his inner nature.

In the course of getting the gossip, he crushed more than a few psychoanalytic dogmas, which took intellectual integrity. When Roazen got into the field in the 1960s, psychoanalysis was at its apogee. Most psychiatry department chairmen were psychoanalysts; most residency programs taught psychiatry almost exclusively through the psychoanalytic lens; and most American psychiatrists practiced psychoanalysis. This psychoanalysis of the Establishment, the mainstream reality of 1960s American psychiatry, was a very orthodox psychoanalysis: it had its supreme leader (Freud), and his appointed or inherited successors (Anna Freud and her circle); it had its institutions (the psychoanalytic institutes), with their myriad (and expensive) rules about how to join the sacred order (a lengthy training analysis after psychiatry residency); it had its sacred writ (the Standard Edition of Freud's works); it even had its heretics (the Jungians, Kleinians, psychosomaticists, and so on). Psychoanalysis was chock-full of dogma—Paul Roazen just had to choose where to start.

Paul called it "Anna Freudianism" because Freud's daughter wielded fiat power in the psychoanalytic movement. He wrote: "In her lifetime Anna constituted an obstacle to research on the history of analysis. That which might or might not have offended her was enough to scare off independent thinking."

Roazen went about the business of identifying some basic historical facts that contradicted orthodox dogma. Orthodox psychoanalysis taught that psychoanalysts should not treat their families: Paul proved that Freud had psychoanalyzed his daughter Anna. Orthodoxy taught that psychoanalysts should maintain a distance from patients, scrupulously being neutral and unemotional, keeping careful therapeutic "boundaries": Paul showed that Freud was very active in his sessions with patients and freely expressed his opinions. As for boundaries, Freud told his patients whom to marry and whom to divorce and even had meals with some of them. The grossest boundary violation is sex with patients: Most early prominent psychoanalysts (like Carl Jung and Ernest Jones) freely crossed this boundary with patients (Freud apparently did not). Orthodoxy claimed that the truth was all important in therapy: Paul showed that Anna Freud and other orthodox leaders had systematically hidden many letters and writings of Freud that contradicted idealized versions of him. A key orthodox dogma was that Freud was almost a saint, brilliant and practically unerring in his wisdom: Paul showed that many key advances in psychoanalytic practice in later years had been prefigured by the detested heretics that Freud had cut off (like Jung's advocacy of, and Sándor Ferenczi's work on, countertransference). Freud's conflict with his student Victor Tausk, and his cold attitude toward Tausk that was implicated in the latter's suicide was a key discovery made by Paul, one that fully destroyed the idealized image of Freud.

Yet while removing the halo around Freud, Paul wasn't a mere critic, but rather something like a loyal opposition:

> Freud was in fact a more interesting figure than the Master whose myth now supports the needs of a bureaucratic movement. . . . It is not surprising when practicing analysts support myths about Freud on behalf of the occupational security of their status quo. . . . Freud can be excused of many mistakes by virtue of his originality and genius. His followers and their critics, however, must share the more standard tests that the rest of us try to live by.

Paul wanted to preserve Freud the man by killing Freud the saint.

But he did so in the interests of removing the dogmas of psychoanalysis and resuscitating its living core.

Paul wanted to preserve Freud the man by killing Freud the saint

---

ROAZEN WAS MUCH INTRIGUED, and more than a bit perplexed, by the passing of psychoanalysis from seats of power in psychiatry in recent years and the rise of biological psychiatry. Although he had been critical of orthodox psychoanalysis during its decades of hegemony, Paul felt that the pendulum was swinging too far, and the perspective that all things are biological wouldn't serve psychiatry well either. Not that he was unwilling to view psychiatry biologically: "I think that no one should talk even metaphorically about insanity without at least some attention to the biochemical side of things."

Paul's critique was about dogmatism more than anything else, and it mattered not whether the dogma was psychoanalysis or biological psychiatry; he knew in his bones that either dogmatism was false: "One of the central problems with modern psychiatry is that the different ideological schools fail to listen to each other. So orthodox analysts have been known to treat patients for decades without turning to any use of drugs. And at the other extreme there are biological psychiatrists who prescribe heavy-duty pills seemingly at the drop of a hat." He was especially critical of the "psychoanalytic ayatollahs" who for so long excommunicated their opponents and brooked no disagreement. He agreed with one critic of the psychoanalytic mainstream that for so long had seen schizophrenia as a problem of poor mothering: "To hold a sick person's hand is a good deed; to go on to proclaim hand-holding as a cure is something else entirely." His conclusion: "zealotry in behalf of any school of thought is likely to produce a new set of follies."

He used to say to me, given my clinical interest in bipolar disorder, "Is lithium really effective?" "Why is everyone getting diagnosed with bipolar disorder these days?" He was willing to accept evidence of some benefit for drugs like lithium, as well as antidepressants or other agents;

and he was willing to accept a reality that some patients had mental illnesses like bipolar disorder or schizophrenia. But he thought psychiatrists were going too far in treating and diagnosing such disorders.

AFTER SOME DISCUSSIONS AND listening to my work on the concept of a bipolar spectrum, Paul asked skeptical probing questions. "Whatever happened to neurotic depression?" he asked me in an e-mail exchange in 2003. "Freud started with the concept of neurosis, and then immediately used the notion of narcissistic neurosis to expand his Empire, in the face of objections from Jung that psychosis was something qualitatively different. . . . Now Americans have naively been starting at the other extreme, and working from psychosis as the central concept, and expanding it to include ghostly entities like so-called Bi-polar II." He felt that something important had been lost in giving up neurosis; that many patients were seen now as having a biological mental illness when in fact they really had neurotic symptoms (of mixed anxiety and depressive content) that reflected real-life stressors, childhood experiences, or other problems of living, not autonomous brain-based disease-entities. He wrote to me in the same e-mail exchange: "Reactive depression is a concept that deserves to live, and I think helps in one's own life as well as understanding those that one lovingly cares for. William James would have understood it I am sure."

He was also skeptical about those who made *DSM* the be-all of nosology:

> Freud used to quote the line from Schiller or somebody, to the effect that a person who does not lose his mind under certain circumstances has no mind to lose. Put that in your *DSM* pipe and smoke it—I do not think anything that *DSM* does or does not say is of any intellectual relevance. . . . *DSM* is a question of what insurance needs require—period. In my view nothing to do with "science," certainly not the life of the mind.

Later he wrote, in his last e-mail to me in September 2005:

> The one point I don't see eye to eye with you on is what I consider the dogma of *DSM*. Its ill effects match the worst of what Freudians were

doing forty-five years ago, when I first started out. The emphasis on hered-
ity and classification puts us back to where we were in 1900. The idea of
reducing people to two decimal points, for purposes of reimbursement by
insurance companies, seems to me a novel form of idiocy. . . . Pluralism is
fine, and for years diagnosis was neglected, but this reification of a scien-
tistic form of mechanistic reasoning is doing a terrible amount of damage.

For all his critique of orthodox psychoanalysis, Paul felt psychiatry was on the wrong track. Biological dogmatism was a twin evil to
its psychoanalytic precursor. And the loss of a place of psychoanalytic
approaches would impoverish psychiatry's ability to deal with the
many problems of living, rather than diseases, that patients bring to
their clinicians. A return to psychoanalytic prowess was not the solution, in his perspective. He seemed most attracted to some kind of
symbiosis along the lines of what had been proposed by Adolf Meyer,
an eclectic coexistence of biological perspectives with psychoanalytic
wisdom. He wrote to me in 2003: "Meyer's notion of reactive types
at least starts with a humane premise, and is anti-pathologizing in its
implications."

WHAT CAN WE LEARN about psychiatry today from Paul Roazen? Psychoanalysis as a dogma should be rejected. Freud as a thinker can be
embraced. Biology as a dogma should be rejected. Medications, carefully used, can be accepted. Not all symptoms are diagnoses; not all
diagnoses are very symptomatic. The concept of neurosis should be
resuscitated: it tells us much about the many people who have psychological symptoms but no psychiatric diseases.

Psychiatry can't be understood separate from its history, and its
history is not a scholastic task, nor a hagiographic one, but rather one
that requires clinical knowledge, combined with historical skill and
training, and, above all, intellectual honesty—the courage to reject the
status quo and to reject one's own wishes. Paul is one of the few intellectuals I have met who combined these qualities.

In an e-mail written about five weeks before his death in the fall
of 2005, after I gave him a book I wrote that tried to understand psy-

chiatry partly based on the philosopher Karl Jaspers, Paul left a final message, again criticizing the *DSM* diagnostic system: "Freud despised American culture for all kinds of reasons, but he was onto something when it came to the ill-effects of pragmatism. Sorry to sound so embattled. I hope to God that Jaspers would despise what is going on now. . . . There is a good reason why young physicians are so reluctant to get into this field now."

With that warning, Paul Roazen left us, much earlier than his friends would have liked, with the German philosopher Karl Jaspers waiting as a final guide.

CHAPTER 14

Karl Jaspers

Keeping Faith

KARL JASPERS WAS A psychiatrist and a philosopher. He is best known among psychiatrists for his classic 1913 text, *General Psychopathology*, where he introduced the concept of empathy to psychiatry, the founding text of existential psychiatry and psychology. He is best known among philosophers as a founding thinker, along with his friend and later nemesis Martin Heidegger, in the then-new philosophy called existentialism. One cannot discuss guides for psychiatry, especially the existential approach, without studying the first and most profound thinker in this field.

I will do so from an angle that has not been discussed in psychiatric writing in the past: Jaspers on science and faith. These ideas are influenced heavily by the late philosopher Leonard Ehrlich, one of Jaspers's students, who taught me a great deal.

Faith is about seeking meaning in life, and the search for meaning begins in an awareness of death. When one becomes a conscious human being, one wonders what the point of this life is if it is to end. Why should we care to live if we are bound to die? What is death anyway? Five-year-old children are conscious enough to ask these questions. Middle-aged adults, who often had not thought about them since they were five themselves, struggle to evade an answer. And the oldest adults ask them once more.

But the question of meaning in life arises not only because of awareness of death; it also grows out of boredom. In young adulthood, when a long vista of life lies ahead and death is an abstract futurity, some wonder what is the point of living; nothing much seems to be happening, people rush to and fro, going to work, shopping, doing errands. Why bother?

Jaspers struggled with these questions because he suffered from a severe chronic lung illness (pulmonary fibrosis); in youth, he had been given a life expectancy of about thirty years. Though he lived into his eighties, he could not exert himself physically; he rarely traveled, for instance, because the mere physical effort would incapacitate him. He also suffered the dark experience of Nazism in midlife. No wonder he thought personal and political considerations are inseparable from philosophy.

He was trained formally in medicine, not philosophy, and experienced, predictably, some of the opposition of academic philosophers to one who was not one of their own. Jaspers, in turn, drew the opposite conclusion: One could not be a philosopher, a *real* philosopher, unless he was not a philosopher. Meaning: unless he was not formally trained in philosophy alone but rather also in the sciences. Why science? There is more than an educational rationale here.

The key distinction in the world of wisdom, according to Jaspers, is between knowledge and faith, between science and philosophy. The parallel terms are more than synonyms. Knowledge is the same thing as science; faith is the same as philosophy. Philosophical faith is, in a sense, a tautology; like saying scientific knowledge. What is unscientific knowledge? Jaspers would say it was nothing. What is nonphilosophical faith? What is faithless philosophy? Jaspers would say it was nothing.

So here we have it: science leads to philosophy; and philosophy is the same as faith. Let's see what this means. Science leads to philosophy because we begin our search for understanding in ourselves and the world around us; we try to gain knowledge. How? Through science we watch, observe, smell, taste, touch; we extend and purify the senses through our scientific experiments: with stethoscopes, microscopes, telescopes; with hypotheses, and tests, and statistics, and measuring probabilities. Science is knowledge, the best knowledge; more, it is knowledge per se.

But science isn't positivism. It isn't positive, absolute knowledge of facts producing complete certainty. In short, science isn't what most of Jaspers's prewar Victorian contemporaries thought, nor is it what most postmodernist critics presume.

Science has its limits; this is trivial now, but Jaspers understood how this apparent weakness is the secret of its strength: "The essence of science is its incompletability; in it, however, the extraordinary fragment counts for more than any—merely apparent—completion." Science is limited because we can only see so far, we can only taste so well, we can only touch so much; but when we know our limits, we see and taste and touch clearly and fully. Science is limited because it is probabilistic, not absolute; because it requires statistics to measure, rather than ignore, error; because it always is a mix of truth and error. Indeed it views truth as corrected error.

HAVING LIMITS IS NOT a problem; it's the solution. All greatness, Goethe wrote, comes from an awareness of one's limits. Jaspers fully understood this wisdom in his great study of psychiatry, *General Psychopathology*, where he discovered that different methods produce different results and that each method has its own strengths and scope— and limits. This is not a limitation of psychiatry; it is the very nature of science, properly understood. Otherwise, science becomes religion, an absolute belief system. It takes some philosophical awareness, in fact, to practice science: "philosophizing brings about an inner attitude that is beneficial to science through the setting of boundaries. . . . The psychopathologist must concern himself with philosophy not because it might teach him something positive as regards his field but because it clears the inner space for the possibilities of knowledge."

None of this means that science is mere opinion, no better knowledge than other fields like literature or religion. Jaspers wasn't Heidegger; he wasn't antiscience. There is a reason why Michel Foucault and the bevy of Parisian postmodernists admired Heidegger fervently, yet avoided Jaspers. Despite valuing Nietzsche and realizing that many of the old rationalist certainties are behind us, Jaspers is no postmodernist. He is too wise for that. Jaspers sees through this "intellectual opportunism" that "is versed in all methods but adheres strictly to none." Jaspers, who saw his onetime friend Heidegger go down this path (and carry much of the Western world with him for the past half century), could hardly be more vociferous in his denunciation of this facile antiscience attitude:

> We have heard the outcry: Science destroys faith. . . . These critics doubt the eternal truth which shines forth in modern science. They deny the dignity of man which is today no longer possible without a scientific attitude. They attack philosophical enlightenment. . . . They turn against liberalism. . . . They attack tolerance as heartless indifference. . . . In short, they . . . advocate philosophical suicide.

Jaspers accepts science as true, as far as it goes, which is very far. Probabilistic knowledge is not relativistic; we can know something with 99.99 percent certainty, and this doesn't mean that one opinion is as good as another, nor that knowledge is merely a reflection of power, nor that money is the base of everything. Some scientific ideas aren't that certain, and others are quite dubious. But with time, science tends to become more and more certain about certain truths, and less and less certain about falsehoods. Over time, science approximates the truth. Nonetheless, there is some room for uncertainty at any point in time, and over time, there are some things that tend to remain uncertain.

DESPITE ALL THESE LIMITS, we have to accept the power of science where it gives us real knowledge. This is quite liberating. If life is full of mysteries and tragedies, it is not unimportant that the number of mysteries and tragedies are today, thankfully, much fewer than they were even in Jaspers's age. In his own medical career, the physician Lewis Thomas eloquently describes the progress of medicine from the preantibiotic era in the 1930s to the postantibiotic era in the 1950s. Where a young boy with a cut finger could die of cellulitis (infection of the skin) in 1935, a boy could be easily cured with penicillin in 1955.

Where children and future presidents were felled with polio routinely in the 1920s, the disease would be prevented by the 1950s. Without modern treatments, like steroids for asthma, it's also probable that the writer of this book wouldn't have been alive to write it. Those postmodernists who disparage science should stop taking their antibiotics and avoid their vaccines in childhood, if they want to be logically consistent. But they are biologically, rather than logically, consistent: they need science to live, but then they live as if science doesn't matter.

So Jaspers accepts science as far as science will take us; and science has taken us very far. Nonetheless, despite its great successes, science has had its failures, and it still has, even in the best circumstances, its limits. It is here that we are left with the mysteries of existence; it is here that philosophy steps in, which is the same thing, in Jaspers's view, as having faith. This is what he means when he comments on Plato's

> *Postmodernists who disparage science should stop taking their antibiotics if they want to be logically consistent*

famous saying that to philosophize is to learn how to die; if this is so, says Jaspers, then "to learn how to live and to learn how to die are one and the same thing."

WHAT ARE SCIENCE'S FAILURES? Two great failures, caused by and leading to the disease of postmodernism, are undeniable. One is the Nazi monster. Nazism was not just totalitarianism; it certainly shared many features with the other totalitarian state: Stalin's Soviet Russia. But Stalin's Marxist ideology differed from Nazism in many ways, most especially in the racist doctrine of Aryan supremacy. The Nazi philosophy was, as the psychiatrist Robert Jay Lifton has shown, a biological politics. The Nazis made a claim to being scientifically up-to-date and simply applying the truths of science to society. This social Darwinist "science" was, of course, a travesty of science, more Herbert Spencer than Charles Darwin; but it had all the trappings of scientific lingo; it spoke the language of science, so it was mistaken for the same. This is the hallmark of pseudoscience, as physicist Richard Feynman has described, and it persists today. But now this pseudoscience manipulates us into taking pills, or not taking them, or believing in certain psychotherapies, or not; at least it doesn't systematically commit genocide or euthanasia. The Nazis took pseudoscience to that logical extreme. Their killings weren't random: they grew, partly, out of an ideology that claimed to represent science as absolute truth. Jaspers knew that science didn't work this way; many of his medical colleagues, being only partially educated about science, didn't. (Physicians were the most likely profession to join the Nazi party; about half of them did; they also supervised and acquiesced, in general, in the Nazi euthanasia of mentally ill people and in the Jewish genocide.)

This was one failure of science: its manipulation by Nazism.

ANOTHER WAS THE REACTION to Nazism: the development of the nuclear bomb. Here is another example of science run amok; humanity literally is able to annihilate itself. Science itself proves it has no morals; it can be used ill or well. Some say nuclear weapons finally forced Japan to end the Second World War. Yet nuclear weapons became a political tool for both sides in the Cold War. After the Soviet Union fell, the impression arose that nuclear war was no longer likely; but recent events in the Middle East have returned nuclear risk to the stage of international conflict. Nuclear weapons continually put the world in jeopardy.

There is no doubt, scientifically or conceptually or politically, that science has its limits. The only question is what these limits mean. As noted earlier, Jaspers did not fall into the postmodernist trap. He knew that the benefits of science have far outweighed its harms; and the future benefits still outweigh future risks, as long as science is properly understood. Science isn't an absolute system of knowledge; it cannot, and should not, be manipulated to such purposes as the Nazis did. Similarly science doesn't produce good by itself; it can equally be used for ill purposes, as with nuclear weapons, literally putting the very existence of humankind in question.

So despite all the strengths and benefits of science, science alone does not solve the problems of humankind. In fact science alone can worsen those problems. The question is what we are to make of ourselves and our world once we reach the limits of science.

ONE REACTION IS TO REFUSE to face the problem. Those who value science may argue that science itself will solve problems that these days seem unsolvable. What appear to be the limits of science today will not seem limiting in the future. This may be, up to a point. But it seems likely that there always will be some limits to science, just as there always have been, although those limits change with time. Those who devalue science may argue that science is so limited that it can be ignored and that the unscientific beliefs of the past should simply be followed. Jaspers avoids both extremes.

He accepts science, and he also accepts its limits, and faces the problem of the limits of science. His solution is philosophy and faith: philosophical faith.

Jaspers famously equates philosophy with *philosophizing*. Philosophy should be treated like a verb, not a noun; a process, not an outcome; a source of insights, not a system; a tool, not a dwelling. When philosophizing, Jaspers is trying to understand what science cannot know. Science can push back the three scourges of mankind—as John Kennedy put it—poverty, disease, and war, but it cannot put them off indefinitely. Suffering and death still happen. And the living, thinking, aware human being—what Jaspers called *Existenz*—faces those tragic realities. And he sees a mystery. Suffering and death, after a while, after all the work of science, cannot be explained. Then all that is left is the mystery. At this point, philosophy and faith begin: Philosophy means knowing that one does not know. It is an ignorant knowledge; or a knowing ignorance.

PHILOSOPHICAL MAN, THE AWARE soul (*Existenz*) rather than the mundane mind (*Dasein*), stands facing this mystery—solemn, silent, serious. He or she has to take a stand. Not taking a stand is not an option for one who philosophizes. He thinks, therefore he suffers. The stand Jaspers takes is to accept such tragic realities, to know that they cannot be wished away. At the same time, such acceptance is not passive nor is it unique.

All humans philosophize; we all try to make sense of mystery. We have what Jaspers calls "ciphers": symbols, myths, beliefs, stories. For some it is the belief in immortality—Heaven or Hell; for others, reincarnation; for others, unity with Nature. Specific ideologies follow in one or another symbolic belief system. Jaspers neither acknowledges nor denies the truth of any single ideology; but, like William James, he passionately defends the right of believing in any one. All he asks is that we fully believe in whatever we believe, while we deeply seek to engage with those who believe in their beliefs. "Communication" is a dry word: "loving struggle" between ideas is more expressive. The philosopher Leonard Ehrlich, who is most responsible for explaining these Jaspersian ideas to English-speaking audiences, interprets Jaspers as saying that truth has a "combative character" that can only be "civilized by love."

There can be no victory or defeat in the realm of philosophizing and faiths, for Jaspers. There are only insights.

JASPERS ARGUES FOR TOLERANCE, but he doesn't do so out of relativism. He doesn't claim that all philosophies or faiths are equal. He clearly values some philosophies more than others. He rejects all specific organized religious ideologies as mistaking the realm of faith for the realm of science. In the world of philosophy and faith, we cannot prove or know truths. If we can prove or know the truth, then we are, by definition, engaging in the work of science. After a certain amount of experience and experiment, if there is still notable doubt, then we don't yet have scientific knowledge. Doubt is the substrate of faith, Ehrlich writes: Faith implies doubt; philosophizing is uncertain, by definition.

Still, one cannot believe in something while at the same time disbelieving in it. Having faith is total, not partial; otherwise it isn't faith. Jaspers thinks that such faith, though passionate and definitive in the personal life of a person, is not necessarily definitive for another person. Each of us can have absolute belief in a faith, he thinks, but only for ourselves; we cannot prescribe such absolute faiths for others. This is because faith isn't knowledge; religion isn't science. Faith involves not knowing, being ignorant, and yet having a "fundamental certainty of Being." This certainty is an individual feeling of an existing person; it isn't something that can be enforced upon another. To paraphrase Ehrlich, there may be many intellectual truths for all of us; but there is only one existential truth for each of us. Jaspers puts it this way: Science involves universally valid truth, but is relative to the methods used. Philosophical truth, or faith, is absolute for the individual who attains it, but it is not universal for others.

Tolerance stems from such individualism of faith. At the same time, we have to be curious about the absolute faiths of others. Though we *believe* in our faith, Jaspers reasons, we don't *know* that our faith is true. So we must wish to understand the faith of another, in case we are wrong and he is right; we must seek to appreciate the faith of another, though we may not in the end accept it. Similarly, the other philosophizer, believing in his absolute faith, will wish to understand ours. This is the loving struggle—not a superficial and optional exercise in tolerance, but a profound and necessary effort to know the truth. Indeed, Jaspers holds that one cannot know the truth just by oneself, or only within one's own faith or tradition. One needs to engage in the loving struggle with another before one can get to truth: "The truth begins with two." Is this what Gandhi meant by *Satyagraha*, the nonviolent struggle for truth? Or what Martin Luther King meant with his nonviolent resistance, where some truth is recognized on both sides of the struggle? The postmodern relativist may seem superficially tolerant; but deep down, he doesn't understand the faith of another; deep down, he devalues it. And the other person, sensing this, will burrow deeper into his fundamentalism. Jaspers says: "It takes faith to understand faith."

KARL JASPERS IS TRYING to promote a notion that is complex and does not easily fit into common molds. He rejects traditional religion and faith, the following of rituals and tradition; one might call it nonspiritual religion. He also rejects simple positivism, or a science as superstition; or its converse, relativistic postmodernism—nonspiritual nonreligion. He also rejects the most common alternative: we might call it the Oprah option—spiritual nonreligion. The Oprah solution, increasingly common, seeks to provide religion without religion. We are taught to practice life, as the clichés have it, "one day at a time," "in the present moment," with a larger awareness of Being, of how everything is connected to everything else. The notion of Karma is there, the feeling that all reaction produces counterreaction, and that good produces good, and evil produces evil. The ego, the self, is blamed for causing harm; quieting the mind, meditation, satisfaction with what one has is recommended. One eats, prays, loves. Many Americans in particular take this course; they reject traditional religion, but they hold on to its accoutrements: belief in God, or some God-like power; a New Age sensibility, with fascination in Eastern mysticism, or supernatural concepts (like extraterrestrial alien life). Cults are the extreme result; a vague spirituality, without much specific content, is more common.

Jaspers seeks another way: he is spiritual, but not in a personal or New Age sense. His God doesn't personally know him; there is no room for miracles; prayer has no object. His God has a more negative content; he represents what science doesn't know; if science expands, his god diminishes accordingly; and yet this god is not small. Jaspers gives that god a large name: the Encompassing, or Transcendence, to give us the sense that divinity represents what is above and beyond and all around us. The analogy to Nature, viewed as a much larger power than ourselves, is hard to avoid. That pantheistic interpretation, so in keeping with the spiritual leanings of the Transcendentalists like Emerson, is not entirely inconsistent with what Jaspers seems to uphold.

With his concept of philosophical faith, Jaspers is trying to get reason and emotion to pull in the same direction. This is not simply liberal Protestantism, a Unitarianism of rational notions, a modern version of Jefferson cutting up the Bible to keep the rational bits and discard the illogical parts. This is a philosophical, rational approach to religion built on, not ignoring, its emotional core. This view is based on the existential realities of despair and equality—that we all suffer and that we do so equally. Despair is the emotional source of spirituality, the need to succor our suffering. Equality is the rational source of tolerance. Our specific responses to suffering are true for us, but we cannot prove their truths to others. We need to allow for the fact that each of us needs a salve for our despair; we dare not take away our neighbor's painkiller, but we needn't take it ourselves, either.

We dare not take away our neighbor's painkiller, but we needn't take it ourselves, either

---

FACED, THROUGHOUT HIS LIFE, with his own personal illness, and, in the middle of his life, with the challenge of Nazism, Karl Jaspers lived a philosophical faith that impresses. He stood up to Nazi evil; he didn't give in; he maintained a belief in true science when science was being misused; he believed in the rights of individuals, in the need for human liberty, when the ruling regime demanded otherwise; he accepted punishment and loss—his job, and threats to his life—without capitulating. He was one of the few intellectual German leaders who could stay in Germany throughout the Nazi era and stand straight and solid for his faith and his philosophy.

And when it was all over, he could speak to Germany about its guilt, and he could speak to the world about its responsibilities. He could fight postmodern nihilism, despite the upsurge in Heidegger's influence. He could discuss the never-ending mysteries of life and death, and he would keep speaking and thinking and philosophizing, without end.

A psychiatry that incorporates the wisdom of Karl Jaspers (and his student, and one of my teachers, Leonard Ehrlich) would be a psychiatry that fully and completely, without any reservation, accepts science. This means biology, including complete reductionistic explanations of some mental illnesses, like schizophrenia or manic-depression. At the same time, it would recognize the limits of science, including the limits of biology for many other mental conditions that are largely non-biological in origin and course, like mild anxiety symptoms occurring in the process of life stress.

In other words, Jaspers practices a *biological existentialism*, a scientific faith, and a skeptical spirituality. He practices Havens's definition of wisdom: holding two opposed opinions in his mind at the same time. Any proper understanding of depression and mania—and anything else in psychiatry—should do the same.

We have finished with our guides, the great existential thinkers of psychiatry and psychology. We are not left with a house, a system of answers, in which to live but rather with a way out. The door is open: We only need to exit.

IV Exit

There are illusions which are both salutary and blessed.

FRIEDRICH NIETZSCHE

CHAPTER 15

The Banality of Normality

IT'S OFTEN PRESUMED THAT mental health is salutary; but we have reached a point in appreciating the meaning of depression and mania where we can say that these abnormal moods are, in many ways, better than normal. Our final thoughts bring us back to what should have been a preliminary question. Is normality good? What do we mean by mental health?

Much of our confusion about mental health (and indirectly mental illness) stems from continued Freudian influence. (It would be as if economists remained confused about the nature of the private market due to the overwhelming influence of Marxists in the financial elite of New York.) Any attempt to explain mental health, therefore, needs to first meet and then resist the hallowed scriptures of psychoanalysis.

The extent to which traditional psychoanalysis has been unhelpful in thinking about these notions becomes clear when one realizes that psychoanalysts are quite confused about mental health. They peer so deeply and intently into the abnormal that even the normal seem abnormal. Their most common view has been that those who seem normal aren't really normal, but rather they suffer from "rigid defense mechanisms": They overly protect themselves from their inner anxieties and instincts such that it only *seems* that they are not very anxious, because "normality is an intellectual defense against anxiety"; it's like putting up an iron wall to pretend there is nothing on the other side. Neurotic folks, more in touch with their anxieties, hide behind porous plaster. Hence Freud's dictum: "Every normal person is only approximately normal."

This psychoanalytic obsession with abnormality was taken to its extreme by Anna Freud and her student, Erik Erikson, who famously identified the adolescent identity crisis as a key to adult development; Erikson went on to identify eight stages in life, from infancy to old age, each of which involved a crisis and overcoming a crisis. Hence the normal course of life involves much crisis. Anna Freud, who specialized in children, insisted that if a person didn't experience an adolescent crisis, he or she would not grow up to become a normal person. Instead such persons would develop "crippling defenses which act as barriers against maturation." As the psychiatrist Roy Grinker (himself a student of Sigmund Freud) said of Anna Freud: "She believes that a steady equilibrium during adolescence is itself abnormal."

Truly the psychoanalytic vision seemed blinded by, as Leston Havens put it well, "a morbid outlook on healthy people."

IT'S CLEAR THAT PSYCHOANALYSIS has trouble with the whole concept of normality. In a century of work—with Freud's Standard Edition collected works numbering almost forty volumes, and probably hundreds of thousands of other papers written by his followers—a search for psychoanalytic wisdom regarding mental health basically leads to an offhanded remark by Freud, who once defined the goal of successful psychoanalytic treatment to be *Arbeiten und Lieben*: to work and to love. For decades, psychoanalysts unconsciously believed

---

"Every normal person is only approximately normal."

---

in this little-stated assumption: if you couldn't work or love well (in jargon, if you had poor social or occupational functioning), then you would be treated with psychoanalysis. Today mainstream psychiatry applies the same approach, though often replacing psychotherapy with medication.

All notions of health, as is well known, have value judgments within them. Clearly the Freudian definition is a bourgeois value: we should want to work, after all; it is natural, and incidentally beneficial to captains of industry and guardians of the gross national product. To

---

All notions of health, as is well known, have value judgments within them

---

love means, typically, to get married; love is monogamous love, and usually heterosexual, producing a family, with the resultant family ties and social benefits of family life. Freud was rather conservative politically and personally, and the mainstream interpretation of his view also has been conservative: psychiatrists have long spoken of the goal of being "well-adjusted" without ever being clear to what one was being adjusted to, and why.

Some have rebelled against the bourgeois content of Freud's definition but kept its bourgeois structure: Working is replaced with "flourishing" (a concept first used by Aristotle to define the nature of happiness), and love is kept, though liberalized to be allowed to be free, sexually liberated, more than heterosexual, and unconnected to marriage and family. If we cannot flourish (find meaning in what we do, have enjoyable hobbies, get pleasure from activities) or love freely (somebody, somehow), then we should be treated, with psychotherapies (of many kinds) or drugs (of many kinds).

This more liberal bourgeois definition attracts but still seems rather unique to our postmodern Western culture. Some have suggested it misses some key features of humanity. The existential psychiatrist Victor Frankl suggests adding, along with work and love, a third aspect: to suffer. Frankl's insight is that much of the meaning that can make us able to work and love grows out of suffering. Since suffering is present in illness, Frankl's view blurs the line between health and illness.

ANOTHER CRITIC OF THE STANDARD Freudian definition was none other than Martin Luther King. In one of his many sermon comments on psychiatric concepts, King explicitly rejected the notion of a "well-adjusted personality." I ask you not to be adjusted, he said, to a reality that deserves to change. The healthy response to an unhealthy world, he argued, was to reject it; and this rejection would be viewed by that world as evidence of illness. Jesus was not a well-adjusted personality, King noted.

Modern derivations of the Freudian tradition, like the psychiatrist George Valliant's concept of "adaptation to life," provide few insights, in my judgment. Valliant has at least done the commendable work, like Grinker, of trying to test psychoanalytic ideas in real-world research. He followed Harvard freshmen for more than five decades and found that subjective happiness was associated with such observable properties as being married and enjoying one's work, confirming the Freudian formula.

He also found that the happiest, healthiest men tend to have a good sense of humor and a realistic approach to the world. These psychological traits probably helped them stay married and progress in their work. Completely normal persons (what Roy Grinker would label as "homoclites"; see below) are Valliant's happily married and working Harvard men. They get along in the world as it is; they are well-adjusted.

When the world rapidly changes, however, in the throes of metamorphosis, normal, mentally healthy, well-adjusted persons are no longer well-adjusted; never having had to adjust to changed circumstances previously, they fail to readjust.

LESTON HAVENS WELL CAPTURES our poor understanding of mental health. He wrote this about a female college student patient:

> I could say she "matured," if I knew what that meant. Often I know what it is supposed to mean: settling for the conventions and expectations of some group, or mastering a set of tasks, such as intimacy or autonomy. But how do we test for such results, when they are so easy to simulate and, more important, are sometimes set aside when a life has different or conflicting purposes. Just as conventions and expectations can fix a lethal straitjacket on individual differences, so standards of health on the basis

of admirable traits ignore the way human situations can call up the need for the most bizarre qualities.

ABOUT HALF A CENTURY ago, Havens's insight was confirmed in the work of psychiatrist Roy Grinker, studying the psychological state of healthy people. In an era of psychoanalytic thinking, Grinker, himself once analyzed by Freud, was a rare breed of hard-nosed researcher; he collected data and tested hypotheses, subjecting psychoanalytic ideas to research. His main focus was psychosomatic medicine (psychological causes for medical illnesses), and he described how, in 1958, he fortuitously found that he needed to study normal individuals as a comparison group for his patients with psychosomatic illnesses. He eventually arranged, through the dean of George Williams College in Chicago, a YMCA-affiliated school, to give psychological tests to half of that small student body (343 persons, 272 being male; they were given four psychological tests of mood, anxiety, and personality). Over two years, Grinker selected sixty-five men as being completely mentally healthy and normal.

These men were felt to screen fully in the middle of the healthy range on those psychological tests, and Grinker then personally interviewed each of them over time. His candor, rare in scientific articles, is striking:

> The impact of those interviews on me was startling! Here was a type of young man I had not met before in my role as a psychiatrist and rarely in my personal life. On the surface they were free form psychotic, neurotic, or disabling personality traits. . . . Perhaps this experience could serve as a tentative definition of "mental health"—its startling impact on a psychiatrist who has devoted most of his professional life to working with people who complain unhappily, suffer from disabling symptoms, and behave self-destructively. Three years after my preliminary shock and after this peculiar population was systematically studied, I came across the following reassuring sentence written by [Harvard psychologist] Henry Murray: "Were an analyst to be confronted by that much-heralded but still miss-

ing specimen—the normal man—he would be struck dumb, for once, through lack of appropriate ideas."

Grinker understood that mental health and concepts of normality had important value judgments, and in his paper he reviews an extensive literature on this topic in psychology, sociology, and philosophy. To avoid misconstrual by the assumptions built into these terms, he searched for another word:

> Because such terms as "normal" and "healthy" are so heavily loaded with value judgments, a neutral word was sought but not found in the English language. Even the Greeks did not have a word for the condition I am describing. Dr. Percival Bailey made the suggestion that, since *heteroclite* means a person deviating from the common rule, the opposite or *homoclite* would designate a person following the common rule. The reader will soon discover that the population to be described is composed of "normal," "healthy," "ordinary," "just plain guys," in fact *homoclites*!

AFTER TWO YEARS of repeated questionnaires, interviews, and observation of behaviors, Grinker concluded that he had isolated the psychological characteristics of the average American male "homoclite," the normal middle-of-the-road typical American human being. Grinker characterized those "just plain guys" as follows (in paraphrase, using Grinker's coinages):

1. Constitutionally sound health from birth on
2. Average intelligence
3. Lower middle class family of origin
4. Early work experience
5. Early strict mostly Protestant religious training
6. Parental discipline firm and fair
7. Satisfactory positive affectionate relationship with both parents
8. Parental agreement and cooperation in child raising
9. Definite and known limitations and boundaries placed on behavior
10. Self-image fair and realistic and achieved without "identity crisis"
11. Mild anxiety, depression, and anger usually evoked by real external events

12. Interested in sports

13. Little introspection

14. Fairly strong impulse control

15. High degree of ethics, morality, and honesty

16. Minimal and infrequent psychopathology

17. Good capacity for adequate human relationships

18. Goal-oriented mainly at maintaining one's current status, rather than ambition to achieve higher status

19. Strong identification with father and father figures

This is the average healthy American Midwestern male.

THIS DISCUSSION OF HOMOCLITES likely brings to mind differing concepts of health and normality. One useful set of definitions is as follows:

> One must distinguish between three concepts: the *norm*, the *normal*, and the *ideal*. The *norm* is an average characterizing the "typical" in a given class or group. It is statistically derived and describes what is—without reference to whether it is good, bad, or indifferent. The *normal* is an expression of a practical ideal which assumes the absence of the pathological. The *ideal* is a theoretical standard of "perfection" which in many instances is a goal to be pursued without expecting to attain it. (all italics in original)

One must distinguish between three concepts: the norm, the normal, *and the* ideal

---

Grinker was writing about the norm and the normal kinds of mental health, as described above. Value judgments are more problematic when we think of ideal mental health. If we can keep these distinctions in mind, we can perhaps best comprehend what the concept of homoclites and mental health have in common.

It's clear that homoclites have little anxiety and depression. Using the standard personality measures, none of the students met the neurotic profile. Assessing neuroticism with his own questionnaire designed specifically for the study, Grinker reported that, in a range of scores from 0 (no neurotic features) to 35 (all neurotic features), only one participant had a score above 14, and the majority scored near zero.

Grinker disproved the psychoanalytic ideology about "normal" adolescent crises. The homoclites in his study had experienced no conflicts in adolescence and yet were psychologically healthy: "The cultural and family background of our subjects was conducive to growth and change without difficulties that precipitate crises or overt conflict. During easy stages of progression from home, church, YMCA, high school, and college, the value systems of their environment remained constant." These boys matured into healthy young men, viewed by all around them as exemplary, without crises.

To BETTER UNDERSTAND THIS conundrum of mental health, we could turn to some of our current knowledge about human personality. I summarize some of it (largely derived from the work of psychiatrist C. Robert Cloninger) as follows:

One is born with a set of genes, which, with the usual experiences of childhood, jell by age 5 or so into a few basic temperament traits. The most commonly cited three traits are: *neuroticism* (the amount of anxiety or sad mood one experiences), *extraversion* (one's sociability), and *openness to experience* (one's curiosity and risk-taking versus risk-aversive traits). The personality theory based on these three traits is called NEO, from the first letters of the salient traits. We all score high or low or, typically, near the middle on each of these three personality traits. Originally based on the work of Hans Eysenck, this personality research has been replicated now for more than fifty years, by many researchers. Among these researchers, Robert Cloninger has suggested new labels and added one more, persistence. He saw the basic traits as *harm avoidance* (like Eysenck's neuroticism), *novelty seeking* (like Eysenck's openness to experience), *reward dependence* (related to Eysenck's extraversion), and *persistence* (being eager or ambitious versus being apathetic and underachieving). Twin studies confirm that these temperaments are about 50 percent heritable by many genes (just as in Eysenck's traits), and that the other 50 percent is predicted by random or specific environmental effects (the usual experiences of life, not the shared environment of family or culture). In other words, these temperament traits are at least one-half biological.

Psychological studies of temperament were usually based on normal populations, typically college students forced to fill out questionnaires in the classes of Professor Eysenck and his disciples. Cloninger was a medical doctor, a psychiatrist, and he began to apply these scales of normal temperament to sick persons, people who were seeing psychiatrists for what is termed "personality disorders." This concept, somewhat controversial, reflects the notion that these persons have difficult ways of behaving; people do not like them; they aren't happy; they suffer from life, have poor relationships, and can't function well. Yet they don't have any identifiable mental disease: they don't have schizophrenia or manic-depressive illness, for instance. Instead, they seem to always have been as they are; it seems to be part of their personality that they are so unhappy and dysfunctional in the world. Many, it seems, also have experienced childhood sexual trauma. Hence the theory that personality disorders grow out of severe childhood trauma (the Freudian view), augmented by some biological predisposition to such an outcome after trauma (the mainstream psychiatry view today).

Applying his temperament test (which Cloninger called the Tridimensional Personality Questionnaire, TPQ; his fourth trait of persistence was added in later studies) to patients with personality disorders, Cloninger found, as expected, that those with personality disorders scored in the extremes of the basic temperament traits. This was a confirmation of the concept: if normal people are in the middle of the curve on each trait, one would expect abnormal people (those with personality disorders) to be at the extremes of the curve on each trait (very high or very low).

As he had hoped, Cloninger found that the TPQ distinguished personality disorders from each other (for instance, antisocial personality characterized by narcissism and legal problems versus borderline personality characterized by low self-esteem and suicidal acts). But he was dejected to find that the TPQ couldn't distinguish those with personality disorders as a whole (all of the varied apparent personality disorders) from the normal population. As he put it: "I was shocked to observe that I could not distinguish my healthy friends from my patients based on temperament alone!"

Temperament, Cloninger concluded, isn't all there is to personality.

TURNING TO THE WORK of philosophers on personality, Cloninger noted a subtle distinction between the concepts of character and temperament. Character reflected one's "personal goals and values." And values are not, in themselves, biological or genetic. This was always the assumption of Freud and his theory, and it was confirmed by twin studies that show that our social and political attitudes are mostly driven by shared environment (culture and family), not primarily by genetics.

So if temperament is driven by genetics and biology and it only partly explains personality, perhaps the other piece is character, driven by culture and family environment. When considering our values, Cloninger decided to model them in terms of how we relate to ourselves (labeled *self-directedness*), how we relate to others (labeled *cooperativeness*), and how we related to the outside world as a whole (labeled *self-transcendence*). He created questionnaire tests for these three dimensions of character and validated them on normal populations. Self-directedness, when high, reflects being responsible and self-accepting and hopeful (versus self-critical and pessimistic); cooperativeness, when high, reflects being empathic and compassionate (versus insensitive and hostile); self-transcendence, when high, reflects being idealistic, faithful, and spiritual (versus practical, skeptical, and materialistic). One can see that now that we are in the realm of values, one is more likely to judge being high or low on these traits as particularly good or bad, unlike temperament (it isn't inherently good or bad to be extraverted versus introverted, for instance).

Combined with temperament, Cloninger's new model is called the Temperament Character Inventory (TCI). Personality as whole, or the self, is seen as "the marriage of temperament and character." Finally, using the TCI scale, Cloninger could distinguish those with personality disorder from his healthy friends.

Yet twin studies of the TCI indicate that even these character dimensions aren't fully or even predominantly caused by environment; they still have some genetic influences. The reach of biology seems never fully avoidable.

ALL THIS WORK—of Eysenck, Erikson, Valliant, Grinker, and Cloninger—has a key implication: What is normal is not within psychological or social control; it is partly biological. Normality, like disease, is a matter of the body, at least in part. And it can be quantified on normal curves, where most of us are in the middle, and a few at the extremes. Being smack dab in the middle of the normal curve for personality traits produces Grinker's homoclites: highly normal people who are highly mediocre. Being at the extremes of personality traits may produce some depression or some mania, and this may be "dysfunctional" in many ways in society and yet super-functional in other ways.

Who can say which is better?

CHAPTER 16

Two O'clock in the Morning

W. H. AUDEN'S POEM, "Memory of Ernst Toller," which he wrote and read at the funeral of a friend who had committed suicide, reminded everyone that they were really grieving for themselves, not only for their dead friend. Each of us goes through life watching our friends and family leave us one by one, and we know that someday, we are headed wherever it is that they ended up.

> We are lived by powers we pretend to understand.
> They arrange our loves; it is they who direct at the end
> The enemy bullet, the sickness, or even the hand.

The shadow of what Auden calls "their to-morrow" hangs over those who mourn. The pall of this shadow is not limited to grieving for the dead: everyone experiences despair over the course of their lives. For some, this despair leads to depression; for others, it leads to death by suicide; many others spend most of their lives trying to deny it and fighting against it by various methods, including the busyness of life or religious belief or materialistic goals. But the suffering still happens to all, and T. S. Eliot's eternal Footman still holds all our coats. So who can be happy in such circumstances? How can life be lived with joy and seen as meaningful?

Not long ago I treated a 25-year-old former ballerina. She had distanced herself from her family and friends, and whenever she was approached by a man with romantic interest, she pulled back. She felt despondent but seemed to prefer her sadness: "I would rather be sad than happy," she explained, "because when I am sad, I know I can't feel any worse." For her, what mattered most was stability, and sadness is a more stable state than happiness. To be happy, one must risk. But it is in the nature of any risk: that it can sometimes fail and that one will feel worse. If you do not risk, you will not fail, but you also cannot succeed.

I explained to her that life without risk is no life at all—that the fear of loss reflected a deep despair which she had not faced directly. I also explained that she was right about happiness. When you are happy, you should know that your happiness is tenuous. If you ignore the thin threads that keep your happiness afloat, you will be surprised to see it drift away under a strong gust of life's pressures. But while tenuous, happiness can still be appreciated. One need not deny oneself the state of being happy simply because one cannot ensure its permanence.

The same holds for being sad. Sadness too is not permanent, and when, deep in the despair that blocks one from seeing any exit, it is well to reflect that the abyss that seems never ending has both a bottom and a way out. Yet to get out of an abyss, one must climb. And the engine that drives the climber is hope.

Despair, unremitting loss of hope, occurs when you no longer believe you can climb.

DESPAIR PRODUCES THE FIRST and main human dilemma: Should I choose to live? Albert Camus once said that the only serious philosophical problem involved judging whether life is truly worth living. He was right because if this question cannot be answered, then no other questions deserve answering. Without solving this problem, nothing else matters. After all, we must first choose to be alive before we can decide how to live.

It might seem obvious: we are, after all, already alive. We do not choose our parents; we do not choose to be born; we simply are born. We found ourselves "thrown" into the world, and only once already there—floundering about—do we seek to find out what we want to do.

Yet the most serious among us question the actual being there as well; they question whether we should allow ourselves to continue existing in this world into which we have been thrown.

So even though we find ourselves alive, we have to will whether or not we wish to continue existing. This is the first and most important problem—and thus the only real philosophical problem (Camus said)—do we wish to live or not?

One cannot avoid the question, because to avoid deciding to live is a decision to *not* commit suicide. Thus, if it is to be a real decision, a decision with *real* impact on our lives, it has to be taken consciously and deliberately. We have to *choose* to live, not simply to allow our lives to continue.

I have seen many severely depressed persons grapple with this question. Sometimes, their wish to die is simply a wish to rid themselves of pain, in their case a psychic pain, which is perhaps the worst kind, since it can neither be drowned in aspirin nor cut out. Often this wish to die is the outcome of our failures, as physicians and as a society, to remove that pain.

THERE IS ANOTHER TYPE of suicide, one that occurs in the impulse of the moment, when one has lost control of one's reason. Usually alcohol or drugs are involved, and such persons will jump off a bridge or shoot themselves impulsively. Had they waited a few minutes, they would not have done it. If they have an illness, they usually are not suffering from an incurable one, and endurance of pain for a limited duration would have led to recovery. Yet these persons do not survive the period of crisis, they do not make it through their episode of pain, not realizing that light awaits at its end. These are the ones we, as physicians, worry about the most, and those we wish to save.

This too is illness, but it is temporary illness, and suicide and death are wrong.

There are persons who do not kill, but rather maim, themselves.

They may do this physically, by cutting their wrists or their skin elsewhere in a superficial manner. They may do this psychologically, by attacking their being from the inside. These people too judge that death is better than life, but they are unwilling to part with life on their own accord. Instead, they damage their life, making it even worse than it naturally would be.

Most persons who fail to find a positive answer to Camus's question fall in this category. Many of us spend our lives psychologically cutting ourselves. We make the negative parts of our lives worse by hindering our ability to live positively.

THERE IS, FINALLY, ANOTHER kind of suicide, one in which the person who commits it remains physically alive. This is psychological suicide, or psychological death. One can die but not cease to be, and one can live but cease to exist. These persons are alive but they do not exist mentally. They live and breathe and talk and move, but their minds are empty, their wills are frozen, and their psyches fail to inhale and exhale. For them, psychological maiming has become permanent, and important parts of them have died. They may no longer have any ambition in life; they may not have any sense of good and evil, of generosity, of care, or of interest.

They are not necessarily sick: their psychological death is not temporary, as in a clinical depression which may last a few months; they are always this way. Something horrible has gone wrong in their lives so that the tender flower that is the self has wilted and died, and still their body goes on living.

Leston Havens comments that many people live this way. They have said no to Camus's question about whether life is worth living, but they have not paired physical death with the end of their souls.

THE ONLY WAY OUT is to choose to live, both physically and mentally. The only solution is to find a way to decide that life is worth living and then to continue to do so physically, which is not hard, but also to make one's psychological world more alive, which is much more difficult.

The philosopher William James grappled with Camus's challenge most directly in his essay: "Is Life Worth Living?" James laid out the logic of the need to choose in life. He said that the choices of life are either important ("momentous") or not, unavoidable ("forced") or not, and viable ("living") or not. For most modern Europeans, the concept that evil spirits take over people's souls is not a viable notion, whereas five hundred years ago, the average European would have viewed that possibility as potentially realistic. We can have consensus on what is momentous and what might be avoidable or not. For instance, most of us have to make a living; thus we need to make decisions about our profession or line of work. Such a decision is both unavoidable and important. Marriage is of similar ilk: most of us need to decide whether and with whom to marry, particularly if we value having children; this is our current cultural context.

So James argued, certain decisions in life must be made; they must be made because they are important, unavoidable, and viable. And if one were to identify these choices, the three basic ones are *to live, to love, and to work*.

We have to choose. The problem then is how to choose—on what grounds of evidence? James's view was that our evidence was insufficient for anything resembling certainty, thus such decisions should not be viewed in the same way as other problems on which greater grounds of evidence exist (such as scientific problems). If we cannot be certain, then we have to choose *despite uncertainty*. This is where many persons, especially in today's scientifically oriented culture, flounder. Today people think that something akin to a scientific approach is the best for all decisions. But there is no scientific approach to marriage, nor to choosing a profession, nor to deciding whether or not to live. So many of us do not choose because we are uncomfortable with uncertainty.

But learning to live is learning to live with uncertainty.

James's genius is this: *Not choosing is choosing*. If we are too uncertain to make any decision, then we have chosen the negative option: we have chosen *not* to marry, we have chosen *no* career, we have chosen to live but without any purpose to our living.

We cannot avoid choosing. To be dramatic, as Jean-Paul Sartre would have it, we are doomed to be free.

Under conditions of uncertainty, James concluded, one can only be pragmatic about one's decisions. One seeks to make those judgments that, in the best lights of one's current knowledge, are likely to lead to the best results. Obviously, one can err, but James sees no other option.

In sum, his argument is that, while one cannot provide definite reasons why one should continue to live, there are many key decisions in life in which one is forced to choose with insufficient evidence. One is forced to choose—that is the essence of human freedom. And one should judge a choice by its results. Life can be worth living, if lived authentically, but not living always has the same outcome.

One is forced to choose—that is the essence of human freedom.

JAMES'S PRAGMATISM MIGHT SEEM unsatisfactory to some readers, but it is not too dissimilar from some advice from Sigmund Freud that I think is more convincing. One day Freud was walking with one of his followers, Theodor Reik, and Reik was consumed with deciding between whether he should pursue a PhD in psychology or whether he should seek to go to medical school and later train in psychiatry. These two very different courses of education each seemed to have differing pros and cons: the PhD took a shorter amount of time and more directly interested him, but at that time most psychoanalysts had MDs and Reik was worried he might not be sufficiently respected without medical training. The options were confusing to him, and he asked Freud for advice.

Freud stopped on the sidewalk in Vienna, held his cane on the ground, and addressed Reik slowly: "When making a decision of minor importance, I have always found it advantageous to consider all the pros and cons. In vital matters, such as the choice of a mate or of a profession, the decision should come from the unconscious, from somewhere within ourselves. In the important decisions of our personal life, we should be governed, I think, by the deep inner needs of our nature."

Thus Freud recommended that we trust our emotions, our instincts, rather than our reason in such decisions. A less cerebral approach produces the best results, despite our not being able to explain why, as James noticed.

And yet sometimes even our instincts can be wrong.

WE MUST MAKE CHOICES in life; sometimes we'll be wrong. To live life, one must choose and fail, and get up again, and fail again, and choose again, and fail again. There is no rule about how many times one must fail before one might succeed to make the success worthwhile. One in two or one in five or one in ten seems optimistic.

But there are no guarantees. Some are lucky, some are unlucky, some risk too much, and some too little. I worry more about those who risk too little, because we start out with so little. We are children, cared for with love as toddlers if we are fortunate, then shepherded through the standard maze of school so we can read and write, and then released into the world. Being alive and able to read and write—these are gifts, but they are not much when compared with what could be: a life full of joys and pleasures and friends and hugs. So we all risk, and we all fail, and we all have to choose whether to get up and risk again.

The necessity of failure has long been recognized. Philosophers of various stripes have concluded that truth is corrected error. If you want to be right, be wrong first. To err is not only human, it is wise. Sometimes our errors can even be planned. Emerson once said that if you would hit the mark, aim a bit above. One cannot be correct all the time, and if one shoots to be exactly correct, one turns out to have missed the mark.

When we fail, we see our failures as reflections on who we are. I, myself, have failed: my *self* has failed. But failures, like successes, do not reflect on who we are as persons. They are events in our lives, not our lives themselves. I, myself, have failed in this activity, on this occasion, or I have succeeded. Either way I am left little changed, because my self changes very slowly if at all.

So not only should we be willing to fail, we should see each failure as a chance to learn how to succeed. What went wrong; what could I have changed; what did I not expect? Failures are chances to answer these questions, so that we can correct our failures and approach success.

"The way in which man approaches his failure," said Karl Jaspers, "determines what he will become."

THERE IS SOMETHING THAT happens in the middle of the night, when you turn around and see nothing but darkness, and you think about how alone you are in the universe, and a deep dread navigates its way up inside you. This is the despair of the night, a despair that summons what Napoleon called two o'clock in the morning courage.

The most hectic person, the most frenzied fellow, deep down, if he wakes up at two in the morning, knows it is dark, and he is alone.

To continue with life in the face of that knowledge requires courage. Courage is the virtue that provides the solution to the problem of despair. To make the choice to live and not commit suicide, to make important choices in life about marriage and work, to accept failures and keep trying—all this requires courage. It is not enough to have reasons to do such things; it is not enough to have knowledge about why it might make sense to live and to make such choices; the real power behind being able to make those choices, the real antidote to despair, is the virtue of courage.

Courage is not an emotion, and it's not a thought. It's a virtue, what Aristotle called a kind of practical reason. It's a mix of emotion and reason,

---

A despair that summons what Napoleon called two o'clock in the morning courage

---

something we learn and are taught as we grow from childhood to adulthood, something we can understand rationally but that we can only enact emotionally and spontaneously. It's something we develop consciously, and once we have it, it's something that comes to us when we need it.

It is this courage that allows us to make the important choices of life. By choosing to live, we take risks, though, and those are two inevitable aspects of living: we make choices and we take risks. We need to accept both realities. Courage allows us to do so.

THERE ARE THOSE WHO, instead of denying despair in return for superficial hope, deny hope in return for unremitting despair. These are the most chronically depressed; the choice is made for them by powers beyond their control; they find themselves in despair and do not know why. They feel too deeply the depth of their aloneness, and they do so not only at two o'clock in the morning but also at two in the afternoon. For them, the reality of death and the passing of things lead to a deep paralysis, an inability to engage at all in daily life. These are wise souls, but they are too wise. They do not have the courage to hope, for it takes a certain grandiosity to believe, despite all the risks, that the gambles of life are worth taking.

People want to live a life without despair. They want to be perennial optimists, with nothing but hope ahead, above, and behind them. Hope is good, but hope cannot be baseless. We are more often wrong than we are right, yet neither should this fact keep us from seeking to be right.

A life without despair would be a life without hope, for hope cannot exist except as an antidote to despair. If you think you never despair, it's probably because you haven't woken up at two o'clock in the morning and looked around. One might think that one could stay asleep, and wake up sensibly at eight, and live life without despair. But the activities of that life, uninformed by two o'clock courage, are mere comings and goings, a series of events that are authored by oneself but could have been authored by others, a reaction to the everyday needs of life without appreciation of the needs of the years and the decades. Before one knows it, in such a life, one is 30 and no longer 20, then 40 and no longer 30, and one's friends have moved, and some have died, and one's parents have grown old, and the streets and buildings are changing, and then, perhaps at age 50, somewhere around two o'clock in the morning, one senses a gnawing unease.

This unrest would seem to be the opposite of happiness—and it is. But if we can hold two opposed ideas in our heads at once, we might see that the two are somehow connected.

ACKNOWLEDGMENTS

When I showed up in his office in Washington, D.C. in the mid-1990s, fresh out of my Harvard training, I hardly imagined how much I had yet to learn about mood illnesses until Fred Goodwin, recently chief of the NIMH, did me the immense favor of taking me under his wing. Not only did he broaden and deepen my clinical and scientific understanding of depression and bipolar illness, he became my constant advisor and guide in the politics of academic psychiatry. Clinically and professionally, I've had no better tutor. Our common roots as Washington, D.C., natives and our feel for the importance of political and social awareness also strengthened our bond. A decade after learning from Fred Goodwin that my Harvard training had taught me only part of what I needed to know about mood, I learned from Athanasios Koukopoulos, of Rome, a great leader of European psychiatry in mood illnesses, that all my American training had still left my knowledge quite incomplete. Through meeting him about a decade ago and attending many of his yearly conferences, I learned new ways of thinking about mood conditions, ideas long existent on the Continent but rarely translated to American ears. For half a century both of these great men, who are friends with each other, have tried to guide their respective nations toward a better understanding of mood illnesses. I hope this work carries on their tradition.

There are some posthumous thanks to be given to old teachers: Leston Havens and Paul Roazen and Leonard Ehrlich, whom I describe in the text. And to others who have recently passed: the psychologist Eugene Taylor, my lifelong instructor about William James, and my first psychiatric mentor from medical school, Dr. Gustavo Corretjer, a great friend who gave me a Latin American feel for our work. I also appreciate the companionship and insights of other teachers and friends over the years who have shared their ideas and challenged me, in agreement and discord, to think harder about mood: Hagop Akiskal, Ross Baldessarini, Charles Bowden, David Healy, Jim Hegarty, Jacob

Katzow, Kenneth Kendler, Peter Kramer, Howard Kushner, Alfred Marguelis, Sivan Mauer, Ed Mendelowitz, Charles Nemeroff, Ronald Pies, Gabriele Sani, Alec Shirzadi, Antonio Vela, Derick Vergne, and Paul Vohringer.

I thank Jackie Wehmueller of the Johns Hopkins University Press for her help and support as editor and Michele Callaghan for her copyediting work. Johns Hopkins published my first sole-authored psychiatric book exactly a decade ago, and I'm grateful that relationship has progressed now to a third.

My family remains my anchor: my father, Kamal Ghaemi, M.D., my mother, Guity Kamali Ghaemi, and especially my wife, Heather, and my children, Valentine and Zane.

Listening to Despair: An Interview by Leston Havens

When I was a psychiatric resident, I observed Leston Havens conduct an interview with a person with depression as part of a special event where residents from the various Harvard residencies gathered for an all-day symposium. The following notes are based on that interview, on January 9, 1993.

Leston Havens strolled in sprightly, touching a middle-aged man by the arm. The patient was informally but cleanly dressed in a blue button-down sweater and gray pants. His brown plastic glasses gave him a white-collar air. We had been told that he was a successful businessman who had taken an Ativan overdose four years ago and was then hospitalized. Something bad had happened at work, where he had been prominent in his field. He had no prior psychiatric care. Havens later said he knew we would like him, since he, like us, was someone who had defined himself by his work; and, once his work failed, he fell into despair.

Havens was dressed in a tweed jacket, gray pants, brown shoes, a blue shirt, and a lavender tie. He sat close to the patient, hands on his knees, his body pulled together, like the patient's body.

While they were sitting down, Havens said:

"I already know one thing about you. You're a good sport—to come here and talk to me. " The patient laughed. Then, Havens said: "So, you've looked into the valley of death, have you?" "Yes, I have." [rapidly] "It's horrible, isn't it?" "Yes it is." "We've all seen it so much; all of us may have even felt it ourselves. It's really terrible. " And then he went on with his description of the patient's despair, constantly also mentioning the strengths and positives in the patient's life that he had been willing to leave behind.

For the next five minutes, Havens talked, with the patient interjecting "yes" here and there and occasional sentences. Havens looked sometimes at him, and sometimes at us, in about equal amounts. He brought us into the conversation: "Believe me, this is the only time you'll ever be asked to talk with a hundred psychiatrists at once. [Pause] But really we've heard a bit about you. [He looks at us.] Here's a man who is successful but who wanted to die. Things must have been really horrible. So bad he wanted to end it all. And he was willing to leave a lot behind: his wife, his work, his kids, probably young kids [The patient's eyes begin to swell], probably too young to understand how terrible things had gotten. Is that right?"

The patient nodded.

Finally, after about ten minutes, the patient himself began to talk more, though still not more than three or four sentences at a time. At one point, he said, in response to Havens's comments that he might be able to have a better life, "I have no values. Looking back on my life, I've been depressed a lot, and I've never had any values. Things have been bad for a while; this was only the last ounce of it. " Havens turned to us: "Well, of course, he has no values. Nothing has value for him. When you're feeling so horrible, nothing can have value. When everything you've spent your life building falls apart, then you lose your values. But we've seen this before, haven't we? Could it be that he could actually have a better life, much better than he's had before, a different life where he could enjoy watching his son at a hockey game, like he said?" "No, I can't see that." Havens turns to him: "Well, of course, you can't see that, because it takes a long time for the nervous system to change its habits. That's why someone needs to hold onto you for a long time until you can see that. You've not had a carefree life; instead you've been careful in everything you do." He turns to us: "Maybe he'll realize someday that he could have another life, a different life, but still a life worth living. But right now, things are so dark, so dark."

After another fifteen minutes, Havens moved his running comments toward the future: "So what is going to happen now?" He asked: "What do you think will happen now?" "I don't know," the patient replied. Havens turned to us: "Ah, here's an honest man. I don't know, he said. He's honest, because of course he doesn't know. Things might not improve. He might stay this way for a long time. He might still want to die. He might do it again. But is there any way we can help him? Can we cure him? Do we know what the matter is? Does he know? Maybe we can help him think about a new life, given everything that's happened. Maybe he'll be stronger after all this, better for it all. Maybe he can go back to his family, his work, his community, where he has been so successful until now, and make things even better." Then suddenly, surprisingly early to me, he thrust out his hand to the patient in a goodbye gesture: "Well, thank you very much for coming today."

The resident treating the patient took him out of the room; the resident later told me that the patient said, as soon as they left: "I'm sorry I let you all down."

Then began our question-and-answer session with Havens.

He began: "The basic idea behind the interview of a depressed man is to show him that you are in contact with his despair and, at the same time, attempt to show some confidence that he can improve. It is difficult to do two opposite things at the same time, but that is our job. We have to be trusting yet utterly skeptical, in touch with despair but confident of change.

"I chose not to ignore that a hundred other people were in the room. The key to the beginning of treatment is to establish a relationship, to form an alliance. That's why I touched him and tried to make him feel comfortable. Your supervisors tell you to say things like, 'So, what does that mean to you?,' but that is only appropriate later in the therapy, when you are on an associative level with the patient, where that is comfortable. But such statements are destructive of the alliance in the early parts of treatment.

"In the physical examination in medicine, most aspects of the patient are healthy. Even when you're deathly sick, most parts of your body work; most of the chemistries are normal. Even when you're six feet under, your hair keeps growing, and your nails keep growing. Only in psychiatry, and this is one of our few weaknesses compared with medicine, do we always emphasize the negative. We say of patients: They have no hallucinations. We don't express it positively. You should cherish your patients' strengths; admire them. That's important. Don't listen to your supervisors, who call it countertransference. You're appreciating the whole person, and not just his pathological parts."

He concluded: "The goal of the first interview is the second interview. Establish a relationship. The rule of the first interview is: Tact—tact—tact. "

After his lecture, the residents began to ask questions. One noted that once during the interview Havens paused for about twenty seconds as he and the patient looked at each other silently. Then the patient began to look down, and Havens began to speak. Asked about that moment, Havens said: "I began to feel his despair more. I felt it more; he didn't say anything in particular. And I wanted to pause so that we both could feel it. I wanted to see how long he could bear it. And he bore it well. He has a lot of inner resources."

When asked why he talked so much during the interview and asked few questions, Havens replied: "I try never to ask a question. Because what do you get when you ask questions? Lies. Of course you do. We're that way too. If someone asks me questions that seem intrusive, I avoid them. But if they ask me reasonable questions, I'll answer them. But intrusive questions get dishonest answers. It is better to make a comment, project it out, and see what associations the patient attaches to it. That way I have some control over it."

When asked about treatment, he replied: "Can you cure him? Of course not. We don't cure anyone. People get better slowly as their central nervous systems adapt to new ways of thinking. The two great discoveries of this century are the understanding of the effect of trauma and the comprehension that the central nervous system has some plasticity, that it is not unchanging. Nonetheless, it does change slowly."

When asked about theories of why this man was depressed, he commented: "You have to prevent your education from removing your capacity to imagine, for part of what education does is to replace imagination with formulations. Hold your formulations lightly, and let your imaginations grow, remembering that all formulations used to be imagination."

A faculty member commented: "You showed him how his view of his life was one of staving off defeat. Another interpretation could be that he feels like a failure despite his successes."

Havens thought a moment and said in conclusion: "The patient feels like you need to win to live. He needs to learn that you can live without winning."

Chapter 1. Lives of Quiet Desperation

page 3, *the premodern, the modern, and the postmodern:* Ashley, *History without a subject*; Kaplan, *Postmodernism and its discontents.*

page 5, *the Superman and the Last Man:* Nietzsche, *Basic writings of Nietzsche.*

page 5, *Last Men, who think they are Supermen:* Bloom, *The closing of the American mind*; Fukuyama, *The end of history and the last man.*

page 5, *Nietzsche writes his thoughts on this topic:* Nietzsche, "Thus spoke Zarathustra," in *The portable Nietzsche.*

page 5, *Behold, I show you the Last Man:* Nietzsche, "Thus spoke Zarathustra," in *The portable Nietzsche,* 129.

page 6, *Nietzsche's version of human history:* Nietzsche, *Basic writings of Nietzsche.*

page 6, *Ubermensch . . . translated "Overman":* Nietzsche, *The portable Nietzsche,* 810.

page 7, *"the Roman Caesar with Christ's soul":* Nietzsche, *Will to power,* 513.

page 7, *Frequently have I laughed:* Nietzsche, "Thus spoke Zarathustra," in *The portable Nietzsche.*

page 8, *taken root throughout Western culture:* Ashley, *History without a subject.*

page 8, *advanced technology was applied to evil purposes:* Bloom, *The closing of the American mind.*

page 8, *the influence of the philosopher Alexandre Kojeve:* Kojeve, *Introduction to the reading of Hegel*; Drury, *Alexandre Kojeve.*

page 8, *Jean-Paul Sartre and Michel Foucault:* Sartre, *Being and nothingness*; Foucault, *Madness and civilization.*

page 8, *There are other perspectives:* Ghaemi, *Concepts of psychiatry*; Ghaemi, *Rise and fall of the biopsychosocial model*; James, *Will to believe*; Jaspers, *Way to wisdom.*

page 8, *works of philosophers like W. V. O. Quine, Daniel Dennett, and others:* Ross, Brook, and Thompson, *Dennett's philosophy*; Quine, *From a logical point of view.*

page 9, *"Postmodernism and Truth":* Dennett, in Postmodernism and truth. In *Proceedings of the Twentieth World Congress of Philosophy*, vol. 8.

page 9, *We all complain about the dullness of life, Emerson taught:* Emerson, "Self-reliance," in *Essays*, 45–88.

page 10, *advise, as Martin Luther King does:* King, "Loving your enemies," in *A knock at midnight.*

page 10, *Thoreau made the diagnosis:* Thoreau, *Walden.*

Chapter 2. The Varieties of Depressive Experience

page 11, *Called congenital anesthesia:* Grahek, *Feeling pain and being in pain*, 7–10.

page 13, *We used to have a name. . ."neurotic depression":* Roth and Kerr, "The concept of neurotic depression."

page 13, *All four of these varieties of depression:* Ghaemi, "Why antidepressants are not antidepressants"; Shorter, *Before Prozac.*

page 15, *let's go back to that old sage, Aristotle:* Aristotle described four types of causes: *material* (the physical substance that makes something what it is), *formal* (the shape of something or its outward form), *efficient* (that which makes something move, or happen), and *final* (the purpose of a thing). In my interpretation, I am focusing on the efficient cause, as the "trigger" of a depression, and the other three causes I would conflate into the idea of a "first" cause—or the underlying susceptibility (often biological) to depression. See Stanford Encyclopedia of Philosophy: http://plato.stanford.edu/entries/aristotle-causality/.

page 15, *For Aristotle, the first cause was the original efficient cause:* "But evidently there is a first principle, and the causes of things are neither an infinite series nor infinitely various in kind. For neither can one thing proceed from another, as from matter, ad infinitum (e.g., flesh from earth, earth from air, air from fire, and so on without stopping), nor can the sources of movement form an endless series (man for instance being acted on by air, air by the sun, the sun by Strife, and so on without limit). Similarly the final causes cannot go on ad infinitum, walking being for the sake of health, this for the sake of happiness, happiness for the sake of something else, and so one thing always for the sake of another. And the case of the essence is similar. For in the case of intermediates, which have a last term and a term prior to them, the prior must be the cause of the later terms. For if we had to say which of the three is the cause, we should say the first; surely not the last, for the final term is the cause of none; nor even the intermediate, for it is the cause only of one. (It makes no difference whether there is one intermediate or more, nor whether they are infinite or finite in number.) But of series which are infinite in this way, and of the infinite in general, all the parts down to that now present are alike intermediates; so that if there is no first there is no cause at all." Aristotle, *Metaphysics*, book II, part II.

page 16, *often repeated by mental health clinicians:* Horwitz and Wakefield, *The loss of sadness.*

page 16, *"let's call it split-brain psychiatry:* Gazzaniga, *The mind's past.*

page 18, *philosopher David Hume noted this fact:* Hume, *Enquiry concerning human understanding.*

page 18, *an exclusion criterion for grief in relation to depression:* Horwitz and Wakefield, *The loss of sadness.*

page 19, *that it proves Freud wrong:* Eaves et al., *Genes, culture, and personality;* Kendler and Prescott, *Genes, environment, and psychopathology.*

page 19, *Mathematical equations can model:* Kendler and Prescott, *Genes, environment, and psychopathology.*

page 21, *a major risk factor for mental illnesses . . . is infection during pregnancy:* Brown, "Prenatal infection as a risk factor for schizophrenia."

page 22, *a large international epidemiological study:* Weissman et al., "Cross-national epidemiology."

page 22, *"Dat Galenus opes":* Temkin, *"On second thought,"* 5.

page 23, *Puritanism is the haunting fear:* Mencken, *A Mencken Chrestomathy,* 624.

page 24, *the hallmark of the disease of depression:* Goodwin and Jamison, *Manic depressive illness.*

page 24, *foundations of twentieth-century psychiatric diagnosis: Emil Kraepelin:* Ghaemi, *Concepts of psychiatry,* 148–52.

page 25, *"Most things in fact are better by the morning":* Thomas, quoted in Edison, *The dark secret of doctors.*

page 25, *In classic experiments:* Alloy and Abramson, "Depressive realism."

Chapter 3. Abnormal Happiness

page 28, *whole recent psychological genre of "happiness studies":* One example is the *Journal of Happiness Studies,* http://www.springer.com/social+sci ences/well-being/journal/10902. The "positive psychology" movement, which propounds this happiness literature, grew out of the initial work of Martin Seligman, and has many current proponents. Also, see, for instance, Seligman's Positive Psychology Center at the University of Pennsylvania, http://www.ppc.sas.upenn.edu/.

page 28, *"extremity to one's friends:"* Lowell, *Interviews and memoirs*, 7.

page 30, *a person with severe depression and another person with mania:* Bruchmuller and Meyer, "Diagnostically irrelevant information."

page 31, *dissertation by the German psychiatrist William Mayer-Gross:* Wolff, "The phenomenology of abnormal happiness."

page 32, *"my feeble frame could sustain":* William James quoted in Wolff, "The phenomenology of abnormal happiness," 300.

page 33, *"make the whole world happy through my own self-sacrifice":* Wolff, "The phenomenology of abnormal happiness, " 302–3.

page 33, Emotions sublimes, *the French psychologist Pierre Janet called it:* Beer, "The nature, causes, and types of ecstasy."

page 33, *"my imagination gave me endless joy":* Wolff, "The phenomenology of abnormal happiness, " 305.

Chapter 4. The Age of Prozac

page 36, *in an "antidepressant era":* Healy, *The antidepressant era.*

page 37, *"today's high-tech capitalism":* Kramer, *Listening to Prozac*, 297.

page 37, *cosmetic psychopharmacology:* Kramer, *Listening to Prozac*, 246.

page 41, *the high use of amphetamine stimulants, like Ritalin:* Many readers will object to the inclusion of Ritalin here; it treats, and decreases, hyperactivity in children, they will argue; it doesn't increase it. Not so. Some children become more hyperactive with Ritalin because they become manic. It has been shown that in adults with bipolar disorder, at least one-third get manic on Ritalin or its analogues. Further, the supposedly "paradoxical" decrease in hyperactivity with stimulants in children may not be paradoxical at all. Amphetamines enhance attention in all people, children or adults, supposedly ill with ADHD or not. Increased attention will tend to keep one from moving around, which is a consequence of distractibility. In other words, amphetamines do not directly reduce hyperactivity; they may indirectly do so by enhancing attention. In many people, though, they directly cause mania, which leads to more hyperactivity. Our research group has summarized the evidence for the above statements in a review paper about the many underappreciated risks of amphetamines like Ritalin, including their clear neurotoxicity; see D. E. Vergne et al., "Adult ADHD and amphetamines."

page 43, *two-thirds of all prescriptions . . . are for antidepressants:* Mojtabai and Olfson, "National trends in psychotropic medication."

page 43, *with cardiology drugs bringing in $18.9 billion:* Herper, "The best-selling drugs in America."

Chapter 5. The Unknown Hippocrates

page 44, *falsely attributed to the Greek physician:* Wootton, *Bad medicine,* 81.

page 45, *rediscovery of the Hippocratic approach:* Ghaemi, "Toward a Hippocratic psychopharmacology."

page 45, *psychiatrists prescribe medications to 82 percent of their patients:* Tanielian et al., "Datapoints."

page 45, *decreased slightly from 71 percent versus 60 percent:* Olfson et al., "National trends in the outpatient treatment of depression."

page 45, *increased from 18 percent to 44 percent:* Olfson et al., "National trends in the outpatient treatment of anxiety disorders."

page 45, *could not identify diagnosis-based indications for such anxiolytics:* Olfson and Pincus, "Use of benzodiazepines."

page 45, *increased from 14 percent . . . in 1987 to 49 percent in 1997:* Olfson et al., "National trends in the use of outpatient psychotherapy."

page 46, *central to psychiatric conditions like mood disorders:* Frank et al., "Three-year outcomes for maintenance therapies."

page 46, *with psychotherapies as adjunctive:* Miklowitz et al., "Psychosocial treatments for bipolar depression."

page 46, *viewed as more effective than either alone:* Keller et al., "A comparison of nefazodone."

page 46, *the biopsychosocial model:* Ghaemi, *The rise and fall of the biopsychosocial model.*

page 46, *while psychotherapies are intermittently provided:* Stone, "Psychotherapy in the managed care health market."

page 46, *only about 50 percent of persons . . . have a diagnosable mental disorder:* Kessler et al., "Prevalence and treatment of mental disorders."

page 46, *"to help, or at least to do no harm":* Jouanna, *Hippocrates.* All discussion about Hippocrates comes from this source, from Suter, "Hippocratic thought," and from Ghaemi, "Toward a Hippocratic psychopharmacology."

page 47, *avoid adding to the burden of illness:* Jouanna, *Hippocrates;* Osler, *Aequanimitas.*

page 48, *"God heals, and the surgeon dresses the wounds":* Coppi, "I dressed your wounds, God healed you."

page 48, *repeated surgical debridement, which delays healing:* Shorter, *Bedside manners.*

page 48, *Philippe Pinel, as a return to Hippocratic methods:* Pinel, *A treatise on insanity.*

page 48, *Pinel overtly viewed himself as Hippocratic:* Goldstein, *Console and classify.*

page 48, *"Millions have perished by her hands":* cited in Holmes, *Currents and counter-currents in medical science,* 13.

page 48, *Rush strongly advocated treating mental illness with extensive bleeding:* Eisenberg, "Furor therapeuticus"; Meyer, "Reevaluation of Benjamin Rush"; Shorter, *A history of psychiatry.*

page 49, *Osler was a cutting-edge scientifically oriented physician:* Bliss, *William Osler;* McHugh, "William Osler and the new psychiatry."

page 49, *based clinical skills on pathological confirmation and laboratory testing:* Bliss, *William Osler;* Malkin, "The influence of William Osler"; McHugh, "William Osler and the new psychiatry."

page 49, *opposing aggressive medication treatment:* Bliss, *William Osler;* McHugh, "William Osler and the new psychiatry."

page 49, *not simply a personal attitude:* Suter, "Hippocratic thought."

page 49, *"he himself not knowing which":* Osler, "Teaching and thinking," in *Aequanimitas,* 121.

page 49, *treatments would arise:* McHugh, *William Osler and the new psychiatry.*

page 50, *"empirics and quacks":* Osler, "Chauvinism in medicine," in *Aequanimitas,* 283.

page 50, *"the great mass of medicines still in general use":* Osler, "Medicine in the nineteenth century," in *Aequanimitas,* 254.

page 51, *he could treat all psychiatric conditions:* personal communication, Jonathan Cole MD, 2005.

page 51, *"inborn craving for medicine":* Osler, "Teaching and thinking," in *Aequanimitas,* 125.

page 51, *"large borderland pharmaceutical houses":* Osler, "Chauvinism in medicine," in *Aequanimitas,* 284–85.

page 51, *"more harm than good is done by medication":* Holmes, *Currents and counter-currents in medical science,* 38.

page 52, *"and all the worse for the fishes":* Holmes, *Currents and counter-currents in medical science,* 38–39.

page 52, *requiring proof of efficacy to market medications:* Leber, "Clinical trials and the regulation of drugs."

page 52, *the more valid scientific proof, the better:* Ghaemi, *Polypharmacy in psychiatry.*

page 53, *evidence of its inefficacy in acute mania:* Pande et al., "Gabapentin in bipolar disorder."

page 53, *leading to an excessive and ineffective polypharmacy:* Ghaemi, *Polypharmacy in psychiatry.*

page 53, *All diagnoses are not created equal:* Surtees and Kendell, "The hierarchy model of psychiatric symptomatology."

Chapter 6. Postmodernism Debunked

page 57, *it is postmodernism:* Unfortunately, there is no basic text that describes and critiques postmodernism completely well. A good source, though, to start, is Ashley, *History without a subject.* Another good cultural source relevant to the United States is Bloom, *Closing of the American mind.* A philosophical critique is Frankfurt, *On bullshit.* An anti-postmodernist history of medicine is Wootton, *Bad medicine.* An extensive historical/philosophical critique is Diggins, *The promise of pragmatism.*

page 57, *allowing for any or all ideas to be defensible:* Dennett, "Postmodernism and truth."

page 57, *but in the life of the mind:* Arendt, *The origins of totalitarianism.*

page 58, *one consequence of postmodernism is eclecticism:* Drury, *Alexandre Kojeve.*

page 59, *as some early critics suggested:* McHugh and Slavney, *The perspectives of psychiatry.*

page 59, *anything goes; nothing is forbidden:* Ghaemi, *The rise and fall of the biopsychosocial model.*

page 60, *There was no science, as George Orwell reminded us:* Orwell, "What is science?"

page 60, *as Allen Bloom persuasively explains:* Bloom, *The closing of the American mind.*

page 61, *George Orwell, so much discussed, so little understood:* Hitchens, *Orwell's victory.*

page 61, *he grieved what he saw as the death of truth:* Orwell, *Homage to Catalonia.*

page 62, *on failure to know what isn't known:* Galbraith, *The great crash: 1929,* 75.

page 63, *"Follow the money":* Abramson, *Overdosed America,* 169.

Chapter 7. Pharmageddon?

page 66, *prominent critic in this vein is the psychiatrist David Healy:* Healy, *The antidepressant era* and *The creation of psychopharmacology.*

page 66, *Healy writes: "Manic-depressive illness provides a compelling symbol"*: Healy, *Mania*, 242.

page 67, *demonstrating lithium's benefits in prevention of suicide and reduction of mortality*: Goodwin and Jamison, *Manic depressive illness*.

page 68, *translations from the original Latin made by European bipolar experts*: Angst and Marneros, "Bipolarity from ancient to modern times."

page 69, *medical records in Kraepelin's Munich clinic*: Jablensky et al., "Kraepelin revisited." There is a common misconception that Kraepelin's main idea was to divide all insanity into schizophrenia and manic-depression (the famous dichotomy). What is not well appreciated is that Kraepelin had a quite clear conception of manic-depression, as one broad mood illness that encompasses all recurrent depression, which is quite different from our current view of "mood disorders," and, further, that a concept of "bipolar disorder" had no place at all in his thinking. It is also commonly thought, incorrectly, that Kraepelin tried to describe schizophrenia in detail. In fact, Kraepelin tried to describe moods in detail rather than focusing on schizophrenia (or dementia praecox as he called it). The field of psychiatry has been obsessed with schizophrenia and depression for more than a century and has paid scant attention (in all aspects: research and treatment) to manic-depression—completely contrary to Kraepelin's emphasis. And, now, even with the weakened and narrow concept of bipolar disorder, some in society and in the mental health professions raise a hue and cry when attention is again given to this long-neglected illness. There appears to be a cultural and professional bias against appreciating and understanding mania and its related presentations in mood illnesses. See, for example, Frances, "The first draft of *DSM-V*; Healy, *Mania*; Paris, *Prescriptions for the mind*; Zimmerman, "Is bipolar disorder undiagnosed?"

page 70, *the narrow nineteenth-century French concept of bipolar disorder*: Goodwin and Jamison, *Manic-depressive illness*; Angst and Marneros, "Bipolarity from ancient to modern times." Unfortunately, there is an overall lack of knowledge about the history of bipolar disorder, not its postmodernist variation, even among psychiatrists. The concept of bipolar disorder can be traced to the mid-nineteenth century in France, when Jules Falret and Jules Baillarger, at the same time in 1854, described a cyclic mood illness that they thought represented a separate disease, definable differently from melancholia. The term "bipolar" grew out of this conception about half a century later, based on the work of the German psychiatrist Karl Kleist and his student Karl Leonhard. Kleist was a student of Carl Wernicke, a central opponent to Kraepelin. Thus, the bipolar concept, far from being the same as Kraepelin's manic-depressive concept, is its exact opposite and has, historically, been proposed and developed by those who opposed Kraepelin's nosology. See Ungvari, "The Wernicke-Kleist-Leonhard school of psychiatry."

page 70, *There it took the approach of the German psychiatrist, Karl Leonhard:* Ungvari, "The Wernicke-Kleist-Leonhard school of psychiatry."

page 70, *not defined by mania but rather recurrence:* Goodwin and Jamison, *Manic depressive illness.* "Manic-depressive insanity . . . includes . . . the whole domain of so-called periodic and circular insanity . . . the greater part of the morbid states termed melancholia . . . [and] certain slight . . . colourings of mood . . . of personal predisposition. In the course of the years I have become more and more convinced that all the above-mentioned states only represent manifestations of a single morbid process." Kraepelin, *Manic-depressive insanity.*

page 71, *such as some supportive genetic, course, and treatment studies:* Goodwin and Jamison, *Manic depressive illness.*

page 71, *broadening of diagnosis in past decades:* Ghaemi et al., "Diagnosing bipolar disorder."

page 71, Healy doesn't cite an extensive underdiagnosis literature: D. J. Smith and Ghaemi: "Is underdiagnosis the main pitfall?"

page 71, *we always ascribe to a philosophy, consciously or unconsciously:* Jaspers, *Way to wisdom.*

page 72, *recently called "pharmageddon":* Healy, *Pharmageddon.*

page 72, *some sense in it comes from Charles Barber:* Barber, *Comfortably numb.*

page 72, *not diagnosable with current mental illnesses:* Kessler et al., "Prevalence and treatment of mental disorders."

page 72, *those who are pro-antidepressant (such as Peter Kramer):* Kramer, *Listening to Prozac* and *Against depression.*

page 72, *versus those who are anti-antidepressant:* Elliott, *White coat, black hat*; Horwitz and Wakefield, *The loss of sadness.*

page 73, *little if any efficacy in neurotic (or mild) depression:* Vohringer and Ghaemi, "Solving the antidepressant efficacy problem."

Chapter 8. Creating Major Depressive Disorder

page 75, *behemoth, major depressive disorder:* Shorter, *Before Prozac.*

page 76, *51 percent positive to 49 percent negative:* Turner, "Selective publication of antidepressant trials."

page 76, *support electroconvulsive therapy (ECT) as the most effective treatment:* Fink and Taylor, "Electroconvulsive therapy." Although the public has been influenced against ECT by culture (such as movies in which it occurs to sympathetic characters), ECT clearly is effective, and, if used with the right populations (such as people who are elderly and medically frail or younger persons who have severe melancholia and marked suicidal risk), and primarily for short-term acute benefit, it is indeed life-saving.

page 77, *a marker of severity:* This is a controversial and unfinished topic. If one accepts that the MDD construct is not scientific or biologically based, then doing so prevents—one might say, dooms—any possibility that biological tests, such as the DST, can detect it. Taylor and Fink, "Restoring melancholia in the classification of mood disorders."

page 77, *French physician Pierre Louis's "numerical method":* Louis is generally seen as the founder of medical statistics. In the early nineteenth century, he most effectively developed the idea of applying new concepts of statistics, applied in the eighteenth century to physics and astronomy, to medicine. He called this approach the "numerical method," despite widespread opposition from clinicians and even researchers. One of Louis's important achievements was his disproof, in famous studies in the 1830s, of the efficacy of bleeding for pneumonia. He was able, by simply counting a few dozen patients and their outcomes, to disprove two millennia of medical "wisdom" and the tradition of the ages. Yet it took three human generations before the profession of medicine gave up bleeding as a therapy. Among Louis's students was Oliver Wendell Holmes, who also had a large influence on William Osler. Shorter, *Bedside manners;* Wootton, *Bad medicine;* Holmes, *Currents and cross-currents in medical science;* Ghaemi, *A clinician's guide to statistics.*

page 77, *a strong case for it, both scientifically and historically:* Ghaemi, "The case for, and against, evidence-based psychiatry" and *A clinician's guide to statistics.*

page 78, *trial of maintenance ECT:* G. E. Smith, "A randomized controlled trial."

page 78, *Athanasios Koukopoulos in Rome and his group:* Koukopoulos and Ghaemi, "The primacy of mania."

Chapter 9. The *DSM* Wars

page 80, *Diagnostic and Statistical Manual of Mental Disorders (DSM):* Published by the American Psychiatric Association, the fifth edition of this manual was published in 2013.

page 80, *International Statistical Classification of Diseases (ICD):* Published by the World Health Organization, this handbook has had ten editions, with the eleventh one planned for 2015.

page 80, *highly criticized by some of the leaders of* DSM-IV: Frances, "*DSM in philosophyland*" and "The first draft of *DSM-V.*" The former involves a dialogue between Frances and many philosophers and psychiatrists, including me, with back and forth comments on multiple papers. For me, that experience was not entirely pleasant, not just in tone, but especially in content: I became convinced, after two decades of naive assumption otherwise, that our *DSM* leaders in psychiatry did not respect science as a primary source of knowledge, and, further, that they explicitly and happily accepted postmodernist ideology as the main basis for *DSM* revisions.

page 81, *laid down in a classic article by Eli Robins and Samuel Guze:* Robins and Guze, "Establishment of diagnostic validity in psychiatric illness."

page 81, *a very large and prospective thirty-year study:* Wicki and Angst, "The Zurich study."

page 82, *underdiagnosed in about 30 to 40 percent of persons:* Ghaemi et al., "Diagnosing bipolar disorder."

page 82, *twice more frequently underdiagnosed than overdiagnosed:* D. J. Smith and Ghaemi, "Is underdiagnosis the main pitfall?"

page 83, *only class whose use has not increased in the past decade:* Mojtabai and Olfson, "National trends in psychotropic medication."

page 83, *scientific evidence is always too limited to stand on its own:* Frances, "*DSM in philosophyland.*"

page 83, *promised that science would have top priority:* I review this history in Ghaemi, *Rise and fall of the biopsychosocial model.*

page 84, *Science matters least:* Frances, "*DSM in philosophyland.*" See also the *Psychology Today* website for discussions on this topic that clarify the underlying anti-science bias of the leadership of *DSM-IV*, such as http://www.psychologytoday.com/blog/dsm5-in-distress/201004/bipolar-ii-revisited-always-take-the-experts-grain-salt.

page 85, *the greatest scientific success in psychiatric history: neurosyphilis:* I have further described the importance of this misunderstood historical example in Ghaemi, "Taking disease seriously."

page 85, *in contrast to MDI and DP:* Shorter, *A history of psychiatry.*

page 85, *the role of the bacterium H. pylori in peptic ulcer disease:* This is another example of why eclectic, postmodernist, biopsychosocial nosology is a failure and has been disproven scientifically. A more extensive discussion of this example can be found in Ghaemi, *Rise and fall of the biopsychosocial model.*

page 87, The Principles and Practice of Medicine, *by William Osler:* To understand the impact of his textbook on internal medicine, see Bliss, *William Osler: A life in medicine.*

Page 87, 2013, *DSM-5:* Has *DSM-5* advanced on prior revisions in the direction of science? I would say it has somewhat but not enough. There are some revisions in *DSM-5* that are based on science and correct past errors based on pragmatism. But there are many aspects of *DSM-5* where decisions have again been made by privileging pragmatism over science. For instance: the addition of a new made-up diagnosis ("disruptive mood dysregulation disorder") with the purely pragmatic goal of opposing the diagnosis of bipolar disorder in children; the refusal to decrease the bloated size of the MDD diagnosis; the addition of mixed features to MDD and bipolar disorder, but with a limited definition of "non-overlapping" mood symptoms (those that are specific to mania, but not depression), which has hardly any scientific evidence for it and is again based on the boogeyman of avoiding bipolar "overdiagnosis." This fear of overdiagnosis is a reflection of stigma against mental illness, I believe, and attempts to avoid overdiagnosis by restricting diagnostic criteria are statistically false and scientifically invalid. See Phelps and Ghaemi, "The mistaken claim of bipolar 'overdiagnosis.' "

page 88, *The idea of pragmatism has an honorable genealogy:* The discussion on this page can have a large number of sources but two references are Diggins, *The promise of pragmatism,* and Menand, *The metaphysical club.*

page 89, *the moral denunciations of this attitude in King's sermons:* King, *A knock at midnight;* "Rediscovering lost values"; King, *Strength to love.*

page 90, *a classic text of medical decision making:* Kassirer et al., *Learning clinical reasoning.*

page 90, *The authors use a Bayesian pragmatic for diagnostic tests:* The Bayesian approach to statistics implies that any fact, or datum, can only be understood in the context of other facts or opinions. So, a fact is situated in the middle between what we already believe or know based on prior facts (called the "prior probability"), and what we then conclude after observing the new fact (called the "posterior probability"). In other words, put simply, facts don't stand alone but are always interpreted in the context of what we previously knew or believed and then they change what we know or believe. This new belief then becomes the context for appreciating or interpreting future facts. Ghaemi, *A clinician's guide to statistics.*

Chapter 10. Victor Frankl

page 93, *what that tragic event meant for human psychology:* While Victor Frankl's *Man's search for meaning* is probably the best-selling psychiatric book ever written and deserves reading, I would also direct readers to his less well-known *The doctor and the soul*, a book of wider scope than his best-seller, which extends and deepens his ideas, collected from notes he kept throughout his Nazi internment.

page 94, *"they accepted dully and indifferently, without seeming to feel them":* Frankl, *The doctor and the soul*, 81.

page 96, *"to be endured where necessary":* Frankl, *The doctor and the soul*, 89.

page 96, *An abnormal reaction to an abnormal circumstance:* Frankl, *Man's search for meaning*, 32.

page 97, *"a capacity for suffering as a possible and necessary task":* Frankl, *Man's search for meaning*, 229.

Chapter 11. Rollo May and Elvin Semrad

page 98, *a human being, a person, an existence, me, you:* May, *The discovery of being* and *Man's search for himself.*

page 99, *we are more often told we are healthy than ill:* Havens, *Learning to be human.*

page 101, *Kierkegaard says, the "dizziness of freedom":* This phrase comes from his work, *The concept of anxiety.*

page 102, *Once Ed Mendelolwitz observed May:* Ed Mendelolwitz, personal communication, 2012.

page 102, *anxiety is not a symptom . . . but an accomplishment:* Frankl, *The doctor and the soul*, 219.

page 103, *such a* biological existentialist: Ghaemi, *The rise and fall of the bio-psychosocial model.*

page 104, *We cannot avoid philosophy:* Frankl, *The doctor and the soul.*

page 104, *The solution is not to ask our philosophy professors to become psycho-therapists:* Marinoff, *Plato, not Prozac!*

page 105, *to use Leston Havens's language, they are psychologically dead:* Havens, *Coming to life.*

page 105, *"characterizes him as a unique and original being":* May, *The discovery of being*, 107.

page 106. *George Orwell meant by his comment that at age 50:* This was reported to be his last notebook entry before he died at age 47. http://www.britannica.com/EBchecked/topic/433643/George-Orwell/433643suppinfo/Supplemental-Information.

page 106, *"what I will be in the immediate future"*: May, *The discovery of being*, 97.

page 108, *based on the ideas of Ludwig Wittgenstein:* Campbell, "Rationality, meaning, and the analysis of delusion."

page 109, *an oral tradition of these stories:* To learn directly from Semrad, read the collection of his sayings, *Semrad: The heart of a therapist.* He never wrote a book.

page 109, *a fictionalized amalgamation of the kind of interviews:* I previously published a version of this fictionalized interview in a blog posting at http://www.psychologytoday.com/blog/mood-swings/200903/no-one-is -psychotic-in-my-presence.

page 110–11, *"Tears never lie in a male. . . some of the things people suffer most from . . . they lose their diagnosis, you know . . . No one is psychotic in my presence":* These aphorisms all come from Semrad, *The heart of a therapist.*

Chapter 12. Leston Havens

page 113, *"holding two apparently irreconcilable positions at once":* Havens, *Safe place*, 24.

page 114, *"Your mother was not an unmitigated blessing":* Havens, *Safe place*, 52.

page 115, *Jaspers called them "life-sustaining lies":* Arendt and Jaspers, *Correspondence*, 531.

page 115, *"He slowed it all down":* Havens, personal communication, 2004.

page 116, *"not moving speeches or penetrating insights":* Havens, *Coming to life*, 71.

page 116, *"a sense of at homeness":* Havens, personal communication, 2002.

page 116, *"cooperative and reliable":* Havens, personal communication, 2002.

page 118, *"different enough to have a separate perspective":* Havens, *Coming to life*, 37. The quote above this comes from Havens, *Coming to life*, 14.

page 119, *"God would speak to just anyone, do you?":* Alex Sabo, personal communication, 2012.

page 123, *"I must be as free and as compliant as I dare":* Havens, *Coming to life*, 119.

page 124, *"Treatment is less a curing than a learning to live":* The three quotations in this paragraph are from Havens, *Coming to life*, 42, 115, and 61.

page 124, *"in which my own effort, too, may be imprisoned":* Havens, *Coming to life*, 205.

page 124, *"Does he get new friends?":* Havens, *Safe place*, 28.

page 124, *"the person inside the patient":* personal communication, Havens, 2004.

page 125, *the patient's existence is the closest substitute:* personal communication, Havens, 2002.

page 127, *"little more than a test of our courage"*: Havens, *Coming to life*, 71.

page 127, *"curious mixture of letting alone and occasionally nudging"*: Havens, *Coming to life*, 205.

page 128, *Les and I wrote about mania in 2005*: Havens and Ghaemi, "Existential despair and bipolar disorder."

page 129, *What has eluded his students is exactly what that greatness was:* I've tried to capture my experience of Leston Havens here, but I encourage readers to get their own experience with his books, all of them, starting with *Approaches to the mind*, his greatest work in my view, and then *A safe place*, *Coming to life*, *Making contact*, and his last work (a Nietzschean collection of aphorisms), *Learning to be human*.

Chapter 13. Paul Roazen

page 130, *Paul Roazen was a central chronicler:* For readers who want direct guidance from Roazen, I recommend *Freud and his followers*.

page 132, *One review of the book was titled "Psychogossip":* New York Times, December 17, 1995.

page 132, *"enough to scare off independent thinking:* Roazen, *The trauma of Freud*, 97.

page 133, *Freud apparently did not:* Roazen, *Freud and his followers*.

page 133, *fully destroyed the idealized image of Freud:* Roazen, *Brother animal*.

page 133, *more standard tests that the rest of us try to live by:* Roazen, *The trauma of Freud*, 246.

page 134, *"some attention to the biochemical side of things":* Roazen, *The trauma of Freud*, 85.

page 134, *"seemingly at the drop of a hat":* Roazen, *The trauma of Freud*, 226.

page 134, *"a cure is something else entirely":* Roazen, *The trauma of Freud*, 255.

page 134, *"likely to produce a new set of follies":* Roazen, *The trauma of Freud*, 256.

page 136, *after I gave him a book I wrote:* Ghaemi, *The concepts of psychiatry*.

Chapter 14. Karl Jaspers

page 138, *first and most profound thinker in this field:* Ghaemi, *The concepts of psychiatry*. To learn directly from Jaspers, who was difficult in his academic writing, I strongly recommend his radio lectures: *Way to wisdom*. After that work, I suggest the highly readable multivolume effort of his final decade, as he tried to make sense of the great thinkers of the past: *The great philosophers*.

page 140, *fragment counts for more than any—merely apparent—completion:* Ehrlich et al., *Karl Jaspers*, 492.

page 140, *"clears the inner space for the possibilities of knowledge"*: Ehrlich et al., *Karl Jaspers*, 19–20.

page 141, *"is versed in all methods but adheres strictly to none"*: Jaspers, *Way to wisdom*, 114.

page 141, *"In short, they . . . advocate philosophical suicide"*: Jaspers, *Way to wisdom*, 91.

page 142, *"to learn how to die are one and the same thing"*: Jaspers, *Way to wisdom*, 126.

page 142, *the psychiatrist Robert Jay Lifton has shown*: Lifton, *The Nazi doctors*.

page's 142–43, *physicist Richard Feynman has described*: See his classic lecture, "Cargo cult science," given in 1974, calteches.library.caltech.edu/3043/1/CargoCult.pdf.

page 143, *the development of the nuclear bomb*: Jaspers, *The atom bomb and the future of man*.

page 144, *His solution is philosophy and faith: philosophical faith*: Ehrlich, *Karl Jaspers*.

page 144, *Philosophy means knowing that one does not know*: Knauss, "Karl Jaspers on philosophy and science," 69–88.

page 145, *truth has a "combative character" that can only be "civilized by love"*: Ehrlich, *Karl Jaspers*, 97.

page 145, *he doesn't do so out of relativism*: Ehrlich, *Karl Jaspers*.

page 145, *Doubt is the substrate of faith, Ehrlich writes*: Ehrlich, *Karl Jaspers*, 23.

page 146, *"fundamental certainty of Being"*: Ehrlich, *Karl Jaspers*, 58.

page 146, *but there is only one existential truth for each of us*: Ehrlich, *Karl Jaspers*, 69.

page 146, *it is not universal for others*: Jaspers, *Way to wisdom*, 162.

page 146, *"The truth begins with two"*: Jaspers, *Way to wisdom*, 124.

page 146, *"It takes faith to understand faith"*: Jaspers quoted in Ehrlich, *Karl Jaspers*, 76.

page 148, *he could speak to Germany about its guilt*: Jaspers, *The question of German guilt*.

Chapter 15. The Banality of Normality

page 151, *"There are illusions which are both salutary and blessed"* Nietzsche, *Thoughts out of season*, 20.

page 153, *"normality is an intellectual defense against anxiety"*: Grinker et al., " 'Mentally healthy' young males."

page 154, *"Every normal person is only approximately normal"*: Grinker et al., " 'Mentally healthy' young males."

page 154, *"crippling defenses which act as barriers against maturation"*: Grinker et al., "'Mentally healthy' young males."

page 154, *"steady equilibrium during adolescence is itself abnormal"*: Grinker et al., "'Mentally healthy' young males."

page 154, *Leston Havens put it well, "a morbid outlook on healthy people"*: Havens, *Safe place*, 41.

page 155, *a third aspect: to suffer*: Frankl, *The doctor and the soul*.

page 155, *one of his many sermon comments on psychiatric concepts*: King, "Transformed nonconformist," *Strength to love*, 21–29.

page 156, *like the psychiatrist George Valliant's concept of "adaptation to life"*: Valliant, *Adaptation to life*.

page's 156–57, *the need for the most bizarre qualities*: Havens, *Safe place*, 28.

page 157, *studying the psychological state of healthy people*: Grinker and Grinker, "'Mentally healthy' young males"; Grinker and Werble, "Mentally healthy young men (homoclites)."

page 159, *One useful set of definitions is*: Bee in Grinker et al., 410; "'Mentally healthy' young males."

page 161, *shared environment of family or culture*: Eaves et al., *Genes, culture, and personality*.

page 162, *"my healthy friends from my patients based on temperament alone!"*: Cloninger, *The science of well-being*, 42.

page 162, *Character reflected one's "personal goals and values"*: Cloninger, *The science of well-being*, 45.

page 162, *driven by shared environment (culture and family), not primarily genetics*: Eaves et al., *Genes, culture, and personality*.

page 162, *"the marriage of temperament and character"*: Cloninger, *The science of well-being*, 45.

page 163, *super-functional in other ways*: Ghaemi, *A first-rate madness*.

Chapter 16. Two O'clock in the Morning

page 164, *T. S. Eliot's eternal Footman*: Eliot, "The love song of J. Alfred Prufrock."

page 165, *Albert Camus once said that the only serious philosophical problem*: Camus, *The myth of Sisyphus*.

page 167, *This is psychological suicide, or psychological death*: Havens, *Coming to life*.

page 167, *many people live this way*: Havens, *Coming to life*.

page 168, *William James grappled with Camus's challenge*: James, "Is life worth living?"

page 170, *"the deep inner needs of our nature"*: Reik, *Listening with the third ear*, vii.

page 171, *"The way in which man approaches his failure"*: Jaspers, *Way to wisdom*, 23.

page 172, *what Napoleon called two o'clock in the morning courage:* The full context follows, as cited by Ralph Waldo Emerson in *Representative men*, 172:

> "As to moral courage, I have rarely met with the two-o-clock-in-the-morning kind: I mean unprepared courage; that which is necessary on an unexpected occasion, and which, in spite of the most unforeseen events, leaves full freedom of judgment and decision."

Abramson, J., 2005. *Overdosed America: The broken promise of American medicine.* HarperCollins, New York.

Adams, H., 1918. *The education of Henry Adams.* Houghton-Mifflin, Boston.

Alloy, L. B., Abramson, L. Y., 1988. Depressive realism: Four theoretical perspectives. In *Cognitive processes in depression,* edited by L. B. Alloy, 223–65. Guilford Press, New York.

American Psychiatric Association, 1980. *The diagnostic and statistical manual of mental disorders,* 3rd ed. American Psychiatric Association, Arlington, VA.

American Psychiatric Association, 1994. *The diagnostic and statistical manual of mental disorders,* 4th ed. American Psychiatric Association, Arlington, VA.

American Psychiatric Association, 2013. *The diagnostic and statistical manual of mental disorders,* 5th ed. American Psychiatric Association, Arlington, VA.

Angell, M., 2005. *The truth about the drug companies: How they deceive us and what to do about it.* Random House, New York.

Angst, J., Marneros, A., 2001. Bipolarity from ancient to modern times: Conception, birth and rebirth. *Journal of Affective Disorders* 67: 3–19.

Arendt, H., 1973. *The origins of totalitarianism.* Harcourt, Brace, and Jovanovich, New York.

Arendt, H., Jaspers, K., 1993. *Correspondence: 1926–1969.* Mariner Books, New York.

Aristotle, 1974. *The ethics of Aristotle: The Nichomachean ethics,* edited by J. A. K. Thomson. Penguin, Harmondsworth, UK.

Aristotle, 2009. *Metaphysics,* translated by W. D. Ross. Nuvision Publications, Sioux City, SD.

Ashley, D., 1997. *History without a subject: The postmodern condition.* Westview Press, Boulder, CO.

Barber, C., 2008. *Comfortably numb: How psychiatry is medicating a nation.* Random House, New York.

Beckett, S., 2011. *The letters of Samuel Beckett: 1941–56,* edited by G. Craig, et. al. Cambridge University Press, Cambridge, UK.

Beer, M. D., 2000. The nature, causes, and types of ecstasy. *Philosophy, Psychiatry, and Psychology* 7: 311–15.

Bliss, M., 1999. *William Osler: A life in medicine.* Oxford University Press, Oxford.

Bloom, A., 1988. *The closing of the American mind.* Simon and Schuster, New York.

Brown, A. S., 2006. Prenatal infection as a risk factor for schizophrenia. *Schizophrenia Bulletin* 32: 200–2.

Bruchmuller, K., Meyer, T. D., 2009. Diagnostically irrelevant information can affect the likelihood of a diagnosis of bipolar disorder. *Journal of Affective Disorders* 116: 148–51.

Camac, C. (Ed.), 1921. *Counsels and ideals: From the writings of Sir William Osler,* 2nd ed. Oxford University Press, Oxford.

Campbell, J., 2001. Rationality, meaning, and the analysis of delusion. *Philosophy, Psychiatry, Psychology* 8: 89–100.

Camus, A., 1991. *The myth of Sisyphus and other essays.* Vintage, New York.

Cloninger, R., 2005. *The science of well-being.* Oxford University Press, Oxford, UK.

Coppi, C., 2005. I dressed your wounds, God healed you: A wounded person's psychology according to Ambroise Pare. *Ostomy Wound Management* 51: 62–64.

Dennett, D., 1992. The self as a center of narrative gravity. In *Self and consciousness: Multiple perspectives,* edited by F. S. Kessel, P. M. Cole, and D. L. Johnson. Erlbaum, Hillsdale, NJ.

Dennett, D., 2000. Postmodernism and truth. In *Proceedings of the Twentieth World Congress of Philosophy,* vol. 8, edited by J. Hintikka, S. Neville, E. Sosa, and A. Olsen. Philosophy Documentation Center, Charlottesville, VA.

Diggins, J. P., 1995. *The promise of pragmatism: Modernism and the crisis of knowledge and authority.* University of Chicago Press, Chicago.

Drury, S., 1994. *Alexandre Kojeve: The roots of postmodern politics.* Macmillan, New York.

Eaves, L., Eysenck, J., Martin, H., 1989. *Genes, culture, and personality: An empirical approach.* Academic Press, London.

Edson, L. 1976. The dark secret of doctors, *New York Times Magazine,* July 4.

Ehrlich, L. (Ed.), 1975. *Karl Jaspers: Philosophy as faith.* University of Massachusetts Press, Amherst, MA.

Ehrlich, E., Ehrlich, L., Pepper, G. (Eds.), 1994. *Karl Jaspers: Basic philosophical writings.* Humanities Press, Atlantic Highlands, NJ.

Eisenberg, L., 2007. Furor therapeuticus: Benjamin Rush and the Philadelphia yellow fever epidemic of 1793. *The American Journal of Psychiatry* 164: 552–55.

Eliot, T. S., 1920. The love song of J. Alfred Prufrock, in *Prufrock and other observations.* Knopf, New York.

Elliott, C., 2010. *White coat, black hat: Adventures on the dark side of medicine.* Beacon Press, New York.

Emerson, R. W., 1850 (2000). *Representative men.* Cornell University Library, Ithaca, NY.

Emerson, R. W., 1883. *Essays: First series.* Houghton-Mifflin, Boston.

Erikson, E., 1968. On the nature of psycho-historical evidence: In search of Gandhi. *Daedalus* 97: 451–76.

Eysenck, H., 1953. *The structure of human personality.* Methuen, London.

Fink, M., Taylor. M. A., 2007. Electroconvulsive therapy: Evidence and challenges. *Journal of the American Medical Association* 298: 330–32.

Foucault, M., 1965 (1988). *Madness and civilization: A history of insanity in the age of reason.* Vintage, New York.

Frances, A., 2010a. *DSM* in philosophyland: Curiouser and curiouser. http://alien.dowling.edu/~cperring/aapp/bulletin.htm.

Frances, A., 2010b. The first draft of *DSM-V. British Medical Journal* 340: c1168.

Frank, E., et al., 1990. Three-year outcomes for maintenance therapies in recurrent depression. *Archives of General Psychiatry* 47: 1093–99.

Frankfurt, H., 2005. *On bullshit.* Princeton University Press, Princeton, NJ.

Frankl, V., 1959 (2000). *Man's search for meaning.* Beacon Press, New York.

Frankl, V., 1973 (1986). *The doctor and the soul.* Random House, New York.

Franklin, B., 1996. *Autobiography.* Dover Books, New York.

Freud, S., 1927. *The future of an illusion.* Hogarth, London.

Fukuyama, F., 2006. *The end of history and the last man.* Simon and Schuster, New York.

Galbraith, J. K., 2009. *The great crash: 1929.* Houghton Mifflin Harcourt, Boston.

Gazzaniga, M. S., 1998. *The mind's past.* University of California Press, Berkeley, CA.

Ghaemi, S. N. (Ed.), 2002. *Polypharmacy in psychiatry.* Marcel Dekker, New York.

Ghaemi, S. N., 2007. *The concepts of psychiatry: A pluralistic approach to the mind and mental illness.* Johns Hopkins University Press, Baltimore.

Ghaemi, S. N., 2008a. Toward a Hippocratic psychopharmacology. *Canadian Journal of Psychiatry* 53: 189–96.

Ghaemi, S. N., 2008b. Why antidepressants are not antidepressants: STEP-BD, STAR*D, and the return of neurotic depression. *Bipolar Disorder* 10: 957–68.

Ghaemi, S. N., 2009a. *The rise and fall of the biopsychosocial model: Reconciling art and science in psychiatry.* Johns Hopkins University Press, Baltimore.

Ghaemi, S. N., 2009b. The case for, and against, evidence-based psychiatry. *Acta Psychiatra Scandinavica* 119: 249–51.

Ghaemi, S. N., 2009c. *A clinician's guide to statistics and epidemiology in mental health: Measuring truth and uncertainty.* Cambridge University Press, Cambridge, UK.

Ghaemi, S. N., 2011. *A first-rate madness: Uncovering the links between mental illness and leadership.* Penguin Press, New York.

Ghaemi, S. N., 2012. Taking disease seriously: Beyond "pragmatic" nosology. In *Philosophical issues in psychiatry,* vol. 2, *Nosology,* edited by K. S. Kendler and J. Parnas. Oxford University Press, Oxford.

Ghaemi, S. N., Boiman, E. E., Goodwin, F. K., 2000. Diagnosing bipolar disorder and the effect of antidepressants: A naturalistic study. *Journal of Clinical Psychiatry* 61: 804–8.

Ghaemi, S. N., Lenox, M. S., Baldessarini, R. J., 2001. Effectiveness and safety of long-term antidepressant treatment in bipolar disorder. *Journal of Clinical Psychiatry* 62: 565–69.

Gillett, G., 2004. *Bioethics in the clinic: Hippocratic reflections.* Johns Hopkins University Press, Baltimore.

Goldstein, S., 2002. *Console and classify: The French psychiatric profession in the nineteenth century.* University of Chicago Press, Chicago.

Goodwin, F. K., Jamison, K. R., 2007. *Manic depressive illness,* 2nd ed. Oxford University Press, Oxford.

Gorky, M., 2001. *My universities.* Penguin, New York.

Grahek, N. 2007. *Feeling pain and being in pain.* MIT Press, Cambridge, MA.

Grinker, R. R., Sr., Grinker, R. R., Jr., Timberlake, J., 1962. "Mentally healthy" young males (homoclites): A study. *Archives of General Psychiatry* 6: 405–53.

Grinker, R. R., Werble, B., 1974. Mentally healthy young men (homoclites) 14 years later. *Archives of General Psychiatry* 30: 701–4.

Havens, L. L., 1973 (1987). *Approaches to the mind: Movement of the psychiatric schools from sects toward science.* Harvard University Press, Cambridge, MA.

Havens, L. L., 1983. *Participant observation.* Aronson, Northvale, NJ.

Havens, L. L., 1986. *Making contact: Uses of language in psychotherapy.* Harvard University Press, Cambridge, MA.

Havens, L. L., 1989. *A safe place.* Harvard University Press, Cambridge, MA.

Havens, L. L., 1993. *Coming to life.* Harvard University Press, Cambridge, MA.

Havens, L. L., 1994. *Learning to be human.* Addison-Wesley, Reading, MA.

Havens, L. L., Ghaemi, S. N., 2005. Existential despair and bipolar disorder: The therapeutic alliance as a mood stabilizer. *American Journal of Psychotherapy* 59: 137–47.

Havens, L. L., Vaillant, G. E., Price, B. H., Goldstein, M., Kim, D., 2001. Soundings: A psychological equivalent of medical percussion. *Harvard Review of Psychiatry* 9: 147–57.

Healy, D., 1998. *The antidepressant era.* Harvard University Press, Cambridge, MA.

Healy, D., 2004. *The creation of psychopharmacology.* Harvard University Press, Cambridge, MA.

Healy, D., 2008. *Mania: A short history of bipolar disorder.* Johns Hopkins University Press, Baltimore.

Healy, D., 2012. *Pharmageddon.* University of California Press, Berkeley.

Herper, M., 2006. The best-selling drugs in America. *Forbes,* February 27.

Hitchens, C., 2003. *Orwell's victory.* Penguin Press, New York.

Holmes, O. W., 1891. *Currents and counter-currents in medical science: Medical essays 1842–1882.* Houghton-Mifflin, Boston.

Horwitz, A., Wakefield, J., 2007. *The loss of sadness: How psychiatry transformed normal sorrow into depressive disorder.* Oxford University Press, Oxford.

Hume, D., 1748 (2008). *An enquiry concerning human understanding.* Oxford University Press, New York.

Jablensky, A., Hugler, H., Von Cranach, M., Kalinov, K., 1993. Kraepelin revisited: A reassessment and statistical analysis of dementia praecox and manic-depressive insanity in 1908. *Psychological Medicine* 23: 843–58.

James, W., 1897 (1956). *The will to believe and other essays in popular philosophy.* Dover Publications, New York.

James, W., 1901 (1958). *The varieties of religious experience.* Mentor Books, New York.

Jamison, K. R., 1995. *An unquiet mind.* Knopf, New York.

Jaspers, K., 1913 (1997). *General psychopathology,* 2 vols. Johns Hopkins University Press, Baltimore.

Jaspers, K., 1947 (2001). *The question of German guilt.* Fordham University Press, New York.

Jaspers, K., 1954 (2003). *Way to wisdom*. Yale University Press, New Haven.

Jaspers K., 1963. *The atom bomb and the future of man*. University of Chicago Press, Chicago.

Jaspers, K., 1995. *The great philosophers*, 4 vols. Houghton Mifflin Harcourt, New York.

Jouanna, J., 1999. *Hippocrates*. Johns Hopkins University Press, Baltimore.

Kaplan, E. A. (Ed.), 1993. *Postmodernism and its discontents: Theories, practices*. Verso, London.

Kassirer, J. P., Wong, J. B., Kopelman, R. I., 2009. *Learning clinical reasoning*. Lippincott, Williams, and Wilkins, Philadelphia.

Keller, M. B., et al., 2000. A comparison of nefazodone, the cognitive behavioral-analysis system of psychotherapy, and their combination for the treatment of chronic depression. *New England Journal of Medicine* 342: 1462–70.

Kendler, K. S., Prescott, C. A., 2006. *Genes, environment, and psychopathology: Understanding the causes of psychiatric and substance use disorders*. Guilford Press, New York.

Kessler, R. C., et al., 2005. Prevalence and treatment of mental disorders, 1990 to 2003. *New England Journal of Medicine* 352: 2515–23.

Khayyam, O., 1983. *The Rubaiyat of Omar Khayyam*. St. Martin's Press, New York.

Kierkegaard, S., 1844 (1981). *The concept of anxiety*. Princeton University Press, Princeton.

King, M. L., 1963 (1981). *Strength to love*. Fortress Press, Philadelphia.

King, M. L., 1998. *A knock at midnight: Inspiration from the great sermons of Martin Luther King Jr*. Hachette Audio, New York.

Knauss, G., 2008. Karl Jaspers on philosophy and science. In *Karl Jaspers's philosophy: Exposition & interpretations*, edited by K. Salamun, G. J. Walters. Humanity Books, Amherst, NY.

Kojeve, A., 1980. *Introduction to the reading of Hegel*. Cornell University Press, Ithaca, NY.

Koukopoulos, A., Ghaemi, S. N., 2009. The primacy of mania: A reconsideration of mood disorders. *European Psychiatry* 24: 125–34.

Kramer, P. D., 1993. *Listening to Prozac*. Viking, New York.

Kramer, P. D., 2006. *Against depression*. Penguin, New York.

Kraepelin, E. *Manic-depressive insanity and paranoia*, translated by Mary Barclay. E. S. Livingstone, Edinburgh.

Leber, P., 2000. Clinical trials and the regulation of drugs. In *Oxford textbook of psychiatry*, 1st ed., edited by M. Gelder, J. Lopez-Ibor, and N. Andersen, 1247–52. Oxford University Press, Oxford.

Lifton, R. J., 1986. *The Nazi doctors*, Basic Books, New York.

Lowell, R., 1988. *Interviews and memoirs,* edited by J. Meyer. University of Michigan Press, Ann Arbor, MI.

MacIntyre, A. C., 1984. *After virtue: A study in moral theory.* University of Notre Dame Press, Notre Dame, IN.

Malkin, H. M., 1977. The influence of William Osler on the development of clinical laboratory medicine in North America. *Annals of Clinical and Laboratory Science* 7: 281–97.

Marguelis, A. M., 1989. *The empathic imagination.* Norton, New York.

Marinoff, L., 1999. *Plato, not Prozac!* HarperCollins, New York.

Martin, E., 2009. *Bipolar expeditions: Mania and depression in American culture.* Princeton University Press, Princeton, NJ.

May, R., 1953 (2009). *Man's search for himself.* Norton, New York.

May, R., 1994. *The discovery of being: Writings in existential psychology.* Norton, New York.

McHugh, P. R., 1987. William Osler and the new psychiatry. *Annals of Internal Medicine* 107: 914–18.

McHugh, P. R., Slavney P. R., 1986. *The perspectives of psychiatry.* Johns Hopkins University Press, Baltimore.

Menand, L., 2002. *The metaphysical club: A story of ideas in America.* Farrar, Strauss, and Giroux, New York.

Mencken, H. L., 1982. *A Mencken Chrestomathy.* Viking, New York.

Meyer, A., 1945. Reevaluation of Benjamin Rush. *The American Journal of Psychiatry* 101: 433–42.

Miklowitz, D. J., et al., 2007. Psychosocial treatments for bipolar depression: A 1-year randomized trial from the Systematic Treatment Enhancement Program. *Archives of General Psychiatry* 64: 419–26.

Mojtabai, R., Olfson, M., 2010. National trends in psychotropic medication polypharmacy in office-based psychiatry. *Archives of General Psychiatry* 67: 26–36.

Nietzsche, F., 1874 (2004). *Thoughts out of season: Part I.* Kessinger Publishing, Whitefish, MT.

Nietzsche, F., 1968. *The will to power,* edited by W. E. Kaufmann. Viking, New York.

Nietzsche, F., 1977. *The portable Nietzsche,* edited by W. E. Kaufmann. Penguin, New York.

Nietzsche, F., 2000. *Basic writings of Nietzsche,* edited by W. E. Kauffman. Random House, New York.

Olfson, M., et al., 2002a. National trends in the outpatient treatment of depression. *JAMA* 287: 203–9.

Olfson, M., et al., 2002b. National trends in the use of outpatient psycho-therapy. *The American Journal of Psychiatry* 159: 1914–20.

Olfson, M., et al., 2004. National trends in the outpatient treatment of anxiety disorders. *Journal of Clinical Psychiatry* 65: 1166–73.

Olfson, M., Pincus, H. A., 1994. Use of benzodiazepines in the community. *Archives of Internal Medicine* 154: 1235–40.

Orwell G., 1945 (1971). What is science? In *The collected essays: Journalism and letters of George Orwell*. Harcourt Trade Publishers, New York.

Orwell, G., 1952. *Homage to Catalonia*. Houghton Mifflin Harcourt, Boston, MA.

Orwell, G., 1958. *Selected writings*. Heinemann, London.

Osler, W., 1932. *Aequanimitas*, 3rd ed. The Blakiston Company, Philadelphia, PA.

Pande, A. C., Crockatt, J. G., Janney, C. A., Werth, J. L., Tsaroucha, G., 2000. Gabapentin in bipolar disorder: A placebo-controlled trial of adjunctive therapy. Gabapentin Bipolar Disorder Study Group. *Bipolar Disorder* 2: 249–55.

Paris, J. 2008. *Prescriptions for the mind: A critical view of contemporary psychiatry*. Oxford University Press, Oxford.

Peirce, C. S., 1905 (1958). What pragmatism is. In *Selected writings*, edited by P. Weiner. Dover Publications, New York.

Phelps, J., Ghaemi, S. N., 2012. The mistaken claim of bipolar overdiagnosis: Solving the false positives problem for DSM-5/ICD-11. *Acta Psychiatrica Scandinavica*. August 17, E-pub ahead of print.

Pinel, P., 1806 (1983). *A treatise on insanity*. Classics of Medicine Library, Birmingham, AL.

Pope, H. G., Jr., Lipinski, J. F., Jr., 1978. Diagnosis in schizophrenia and manic-depressive illness: A reassessment of the specificity of "schizophrenic" symptoms in the light of current research. *Archives of General Psychiatry* 35, 811–28.

Quine, W. V. O., 1980 (1953). *From a logical point of view: Nine logico-philosophical essays*, 2nd rev. ed. Harvard University Press, Cambridge, MA.

Reik, T., 1948 (1998). *Listening with the third ear*. Farrar, Straus, and Giroux, New York.

Roazen, P., 1969. *Brother animal: The story of Freud and Tausk*. Knopf, New York.

Roazen, P., 1992a. *Freud and his followers*. Da Capo Press, New York.

Roazen, P., 1992b. *The trauma of Freud*. Transaction Publishers, Brunswick, NJ.

Roazen, P., 1995. *How Freud worked: First-hand accounts of his patients*. Aronson, Northvale, NJ.

Roazen, P., 1997. Finding oneself in exile. *Queen's Quarterly* 104: 404–13.

Robins, E. and Guze, S. B., 1970. Establishment of diagnostic validity in psychiatric illness: Its application to schizophrenia. *American Journal of Psychiatry* 126: 983–87.

Ross, D., Brook A., Thompson, D., 2000. *Dennett's philosophy: A comprehensive assessment*. MIT Press, Cambridge, MA.

Roth, M., Kerr, T., 1994. The concept of neurotic depression: A plea for reinstatement. In *The clinical approach in psychiatry*, edited by P. Pichot, W. Rein. Synthelabo, Paris.

Salvatore, P., et al., 2002. Weygandt's *On the mixed states of manic-depressive insanity*: A translation and commentary on its significance in the evolution of the concept of bipolar disorder. *Harvard Review of Psychiatry* 10: 255–75.

Sartre, J.-P., 2001. *Being and nothingness*. Citadel, New York.

Semrad, E., 1984. *Semrad: The heart of a therapist*. Aronson, Northvale, NJ.

Shorter, E., 1985. *Bedside manners*. Simon and Schuster, New York.

Shorter, E., 1997. *A history of psychiatry*. Wiley, New York.

Shorter, E., 2009. *Before Prozac: The troubled history of mood disorders in psychiatry*. Oxford University Press, New York.

Simon, N. M., et al., 2004. Anxiety disorder comorbidity in bipolar disorder patients: Data from the first 500 participants in the Systematic Treatment Enhancement Program for Bipolar Disorder (STEP-BD). *American Journal of Psychiatry* 161: 2222–29.

Smith, D. J., Ghaemi, S. N., 2010. Is underdiagnosis the main pitfall when diagnosing bipolar disorder? Yes. *British Medical Journal* 340: c854.

Smith, G. E., 2010. A randomized controlled trial comparing the memory effects of continuation electroconvulsive therapy versus continuation pharmacotherapy: Results from the Consortium for Research in ECT (CORE) study. *Journal of Clinical Psychiatry* 71: 185–93.

Smith, S. (Ed.), 1985. *Twentieth century poetry*. St. James Press, Farmington Hills, MI.

Stone, A. A., 2001. "Psychotherapy in the managed care health market." *Journal of Psychiatric Practice* 7: 238–43.

Sullivan, H. S., 1940 (1953). *Conceptions of modern psychiatry*. Norton, New York.

Sullivan, H. S., 1954. *The psychiatric interview*. Norton, New York.

Surtees, P. G., Kendell, R. E., 1979. The hierarchy model of psychiatric symptomatology: An investigation based on present state examination ratings. *British Journal of Psychiatry* 135: 438–43.

Suter, R. E., 1988. Hippocratic thought: Its relationship to and between Andrew Taylor Still and Sir William Osler. *Journal of the American Osteopathic Association* 88: 1243–46, 1249–54.

Tanielian, T. L., et al., 2001. Datapoints: Trends in psychiatric practice, 1988–1998: II. Caseload and treatment characteristics. *Psychiatric Services* 52: 880.

Taylor, M. A., Fink, M., 2008. Restoring melancholia in the classification of mood disorders. *Journal of Affective Disorders* 105: 1–14.

Temkin, O., 2002. *"On second thought" and other essays in the history of medicine.* Johns Hopkins Press, Baltimore.

Thomas, L., 1995. *The youngest science: Notes of a medicine-watcher.* Penguin Press, New York.

Thoreau, H. D., 1854 (2004). *Walden.* Yale University Press, New Haven.

Tillich, P., 2000. *The courage to be.* Yale University Press, New Haven.

Turner, E. H., et al., 2008. Selective publication of antidepressant trials and its influence on apparent efficacy. *New England Journal of Medicine* 358: 252–60.

Ungvari, G. S., 1993. The Wernicke-Kleist-Leonhard school of psychiatry. *Biological Psychiatry* 34: 749–52.

Valliant, G. E., 1977. *Adaptation to life.* Little, Brown, Boston.

Vergne, D. E., Whitham, E. A., Barroilhet, S., Fradkin, Y., Ghaemi, S. N., 2011. Adult ADHD and amphetamines: A new paradigm. *Neuropsychiatry* 1: 591–98.

Vohringer, P. A., Ghaemi, S. N., 2011. Solving the antidepressant efficacy problem: Effect sizes in major depressive disorder. *Clinical Therapeutics,* 33: B49–B61.

Weissman, M. M., et al., 1996. Cross-national epidemiology of major depression and bipolar disorder. *JAMA* 276: 293–99.

Wicki, W., Angst, J., 1991. The Zurich Study. X. Hypomania in a 28- to 30-year-old cohort. *European Archives of Psychiatry and Clinical Neuroscience* 240: 339–48.

Wilbur, R., 1989. *New and collected poems.* Mariner Books, New York.

Winnicott, D., 1986. *Home is where we start from: Essays by a psychoanalyst.* Norton, New York.

Wolff, S., 2000. The phenomenology of abnormal happiness: A translation from the German of William Mayer-Gross's doctoral thesis. *Philosophy, Psychiatry, & Psychology* 7: 295–306.

Wootton, D., 2006. *Bad medicine: Doctors doing harm since Hippocrates.* Oxford University Press, Oxford.

World Health Organization, 1990. *International classification of diseases and related health problems,* 10th ed. World Health Organization, Geneva, Switzerland.

Zimmerman, M., Ruggero, C. J., Chelminski, I., Young, D. 2008. Is bipolar disorder overdiagnosed? *Journal of Clinical Psychiatry* 69(6): 935–40.